They say that life is a marathon, not a sprint. To Dave Skattum that is literally true. After transforming himself from a middle-aged couch potato into a physically, emotionally and spiritually fit man, Dave shares with you the lessons he learned in a practical, informative and light-hearted way. I highly recommend *The 4 Pillars of Men's Health*.

—*Henry Kriegel, Talk Show Host/Activist*

I've known Dave for 25 years and have witnessed an amazing transformation in him spiritually, mentally and physically as he has personally applied the principles and lifestyle changes that he shares in this book. If you are serious about improving the quality of your life and moving your relationships to a higher level, I recommend that you read Dave's story and follow his advice. It will motivate and challenge you to make positive changes in your life.

—*Dr. Duane Huie, Pastor at Livingston Christian Center*

The 4 Pillars of Men's Health captures the reality of the majority of men's-health issues these days. As a health-care provider, I am often asked what are the most important components of health. These four pillars hit the nail on the head! These life-changing steps towards health are not thrown at you like a fad diet that will never last. Slow and steady wins the race. Taking these steps gradually, keeping your eyes on the ultimate goal, will help you achieve better health. Dave's four pillars are fun but also powerful. They will undoubtedly have a major effect on starting or continuing on your road to great health.

—*Dustin Rising, D.C., GallatinValleyChiropractic.com*

Dave nails it with his four pillars—simple-to-read, easy-to-understand and fun. This book isn't like all the other junk out there that teaches you to LOOK healthy; instead, it teaches you how to BE healthy. This is a new go-to resource especially for men looking to make a change like Dave did. You can sit around and hope for your health to improve, or join Dave on his journey to master your health today!

—*Peter Frumenti, Owner at OnlineSalesTeam6.com*

Dave is a downright guru when it comes to getting healthy and feeling great. This book will leave you with the tools you need to feel better, get fit, have more energy, and improve your life on all levels. Take action and pick up this book so you can get on the fast track to feeling like a million bucks!

—*Pete Sveen, Owner at DIYPete.com*

The 4 Pillars of Men's Health feels like unpretentious and honest advice from a trusted friend. It is packed with simple yet powerful and eye-opening concepts that will help you live a truly fulfilled and healthy life. His relaxed writing makes you not want to put it down until the very end. Buy a copy for yourself and buy a few for gifts for those men around you who are ready to improve the quality of their lives.

—*Sunny Faronbi, President of Rehoboth Consulting, Inc.*

In the last few years I've personally watched as Dave has embraced everything in this book and changed his life. If you truly want to change, the tools he is offering are simple, but they require you to buckle up and do them. The best part is that Dave is speaking from his own experience and I promise you he's lived it. Dave has run hundreds of miles, biked thousands of miles, and swam over a hundred miles. The transformation didn't end there—his energy, great attitude, and quality of life have gone through the roof. Ask anyone who knows him.

—*Joe Lair, Motivational Speaker*

So proud of my husband for the positive changes that he has made—such a difference! It's been surprising how he has changed the way he thinks about food, making a total turnaround from unhealthy to healthy choices. As a healthy eater myself, I was so pleased. The only problem is now I have to share my kitchen! These changes have made such a wonderful difference in our family's lives.

—*Laurie Skattum, Dave's wife*

The 4 Pillars of Men's Health

Resources for Restoring Vigor and Vitality

Dave Skattum

PINE CREEK
PUBLISHING HOUSE

The 4 Pillars of Men's Health
Resources for Restoring Vigor and Vitality
by Dave Skattum

Copyright © 2018 by Dave Skattum
and Pine Creek Publishing House

Print ISBN: 978-0-9994988-0-4
Ebook ISBN: 978-0-9994988-1-1

Published by
PINE CREEK PUBLISHING HOUSE
P.O. Box 833
Livingston • Montana 59047

Printed in the United States of America

Foreword by Dr. Benjamin N. Flook
Editing, graphics and layout by Denis Ouellette

More information, addition copies and formats, visit:
The4PillarsOfMensHealth.com

I dedicate this book
to my wife, Laurie, and to my kids—
Josh, Heidi and Jordan.

I love you guys!

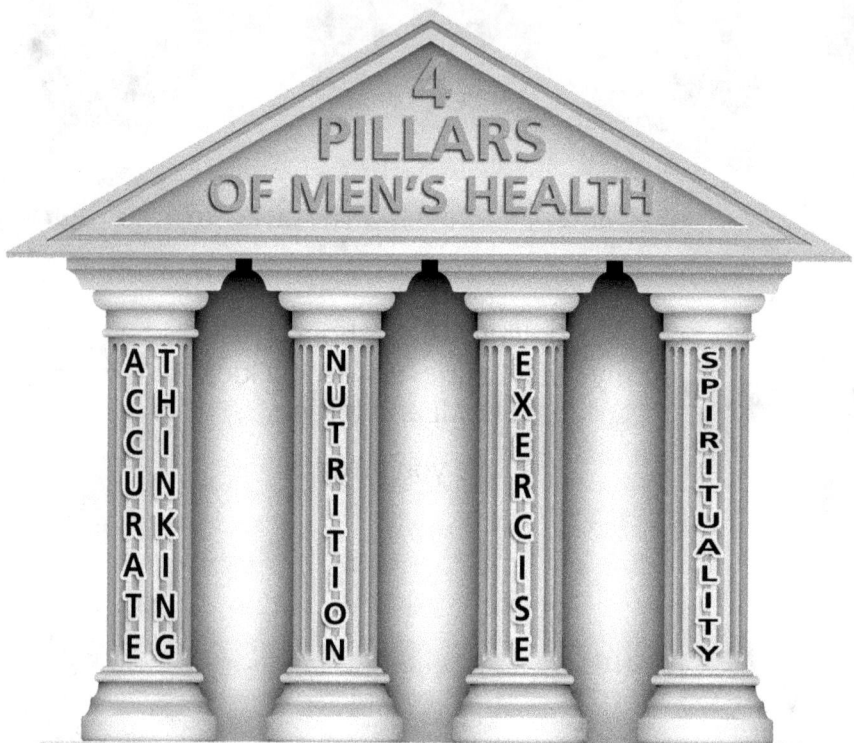

4
PILLARS
OF MEN'S HEALTH

ACCURATE THINKING

NUTRITION

EXERCISE

SPIRITUALITY

The4PillarsOfMensHealth.com
Resources for Restoring Vigor & Vitality

CONTENTS

Foreword

As the health-science researcher Myron Wentz would say, "We are living too short and dying too long." He is referring to the burden of chronic, degenerative disease that afflicts most of us at some point in our lives— this includes cancer, arthritis, diabetes, obesity, and heart disease. What are the main factors that drive these conditions? Can anything be done to reverse and, better yet, prevent this epidemic of disease? Spoiler alert: the answers await you in this book by my good friend and associate, Dave Skattum.

As a family-practice physician here in Livingston, MT, most of the people I see come in with the idea that the treatment they are going to receive is going to "fix their problem" and keep them healthy. In reality, though, we are often managing symptoms and, at best, slowing the progression of the disease process. The medications and other treatments we offer are not the solution to long-term health and vitality. Then what is? It's only when people become motivated and acquire the tools and resources to turn their often deeply ingrained habits around that real progress toward health can be made. That's where Dave's four pillars come in.

Certainly, a large part of staying healthy or recovering one's health, if it's lost or declining, is through a nutritious diet and regular exercise, but can these two pillars alone hold up your temple? Always going for the big picture, Dave discovered through personal experience that in order to change one's outer habits, one's inner life must also be addressed. Never one to avoid the big questions, Dave examines and makes easy that inner world of one's thoughts and one's relationship with the Divine. I am excited that Dave has presented such an entertaining, practical and inspirational book to help us sort through these four key areas of health.

Dave wouldn't mind me saying that he was not the picture of health when I first met him about 15 years ago, and over the next several years, things only got worse. I was genuinely worried for him as I could see his waistline expanding and his energy levels declining. So how is it that this hard-working, busy man, on a fast track to major health problems, was able to turn things around? How did he get from an over-the-hill, middle-age slump to running over the Absaroka Mountain trails with his two sons, one age 30 and the other a teenager? Read on and find out!

Dave is not a patient of mine. He improved his health neither by medications nor by following the latest health kick or fad diet. He accomplished it by seeking out and then applying timeless principles that complement how we are created, and by tapping into his innate, natural ability to self-heal. Dave and I are active in the same local church, and our sons attend Summit Christian Academy, a small private school we helped start. The four pillars that Dave would have us subscribe to have their foundations in scripture and in good-old common sense. We believe that following the Word of God goes hand in hand with the principles laid down by Mother Nature, from which our bodies were made.

Dave started off with not much more than a leap of faith. You will learn along with him and hopefully you will be motivated to join him in reshaping not only your body, but your soul as well. Get ready for the four pillars and enjoy the journey!

—*Benjamin N. Flook, MD,*
  Livingston Healthcare

Acknowledgements

Ahuge project like this requires more than I could ever accomplish on my own. There are so many people who have impacted my life and way of thinking. Thank you all so much!

I am especially grateful to a few team members without whom this book would not have come into being:

- My editor, graphic designer, and all-around healthy guy, Denis Ouellette
- Dr. Joel Fuhrman, who helped me change my nutrition habits and trained me as a Nutritarian
- My pastor, Dr. Duane Huie, who believed in me a long time ago, and with whom I built a thriving children's ministry
- My parents, Dennis and Lou Ann Skattum, who toughened me up and are always supportive
- Toastmasters International and my local Toastmasters friends who gave me a platform to build upon
- Everyone who proofed this work and supplied their great feedback

Of course, I would be nowhere without my faith and hope in my Creator. St. Paul admonished to the Romans: *Do not conform to the patterns of this world, but be transformed by the renewing of your mind* and to that I'll add: the renewing of your body!

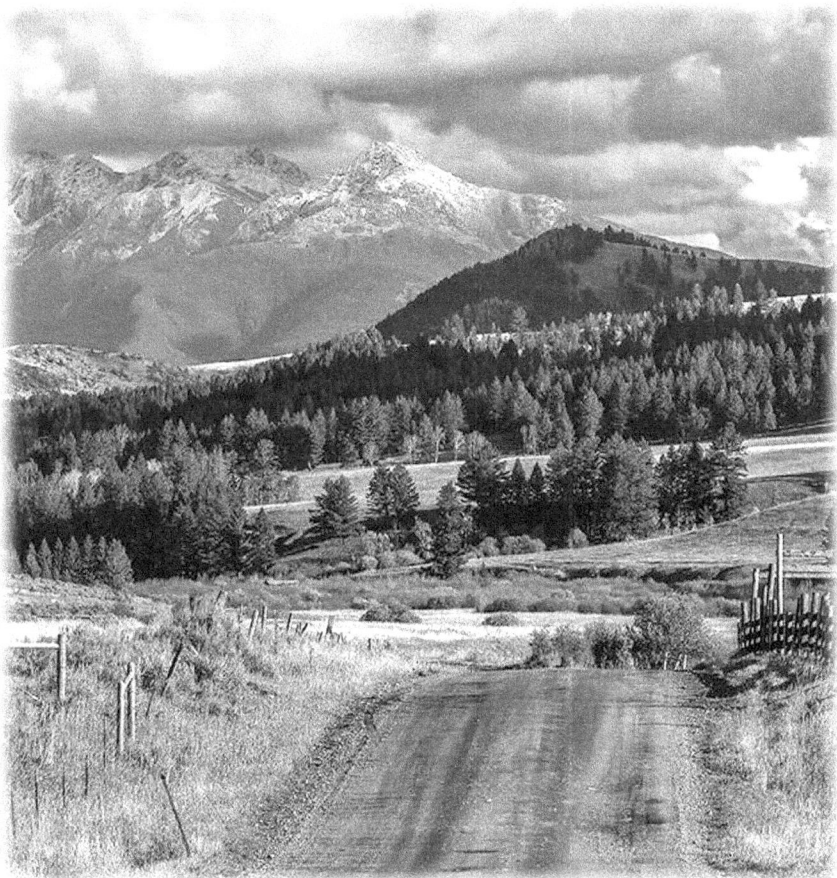

Photo by Jim Harrison

Approaching the Absaroka-Beartooth Wilderness
along a country road in Paradise Valley, Montana,
where Dave and his sons love to bike and run.
Follow their adventures at Run723.com.

Introduction

*We keep moving forward, opening new doors
and doing new things, because we're curious,
and curiosity keeps leading us
down new paths.*

—Walt Disney

In my late forties, I saw some of my friends suffering from some horrible health situations and I started to watch my knees getting weaker and my belly getting bigger. I knew my friends were suffering from choices they had made in their earlier life and I knew I was on the same path to destruction.

I made changes in my eating choices, my sedentary lifestyle and my "stinking thinking." I renewed my spiritual life. I call this support system my four pillars because they really do hold up my life. As I found, if each pillar is healthy, our lives will be happier and more exciting and fulfilling. The Four Pillars we'll explore in detail are:

1) **Accurate Thinking**—We must choose to look at life from a positive angle, with accurate thought.

2) **Nutrition**—The food we eat impacts not only how we feel right after a meal; it also impacts our bodies' ability to function at a high level and to live long and stay healthy.

3) **Exercise**—Keeping our body in shape gives us energy to be strong and achieve our goals.

4) **Spirituality**—Being tuned in spiritually helps us discover our life's mission and live it out, and connects us to the next life.

Discovering these pillars has been an exciting journey. I have been shocked by the results and transformations that I've seen in my life. I got so excited about the things I learned, I decided to write them down for you, so you can find the satisfaction and joy that I found.

Each of us is at a different place in life. Some areas we have mastered, while others we might be floundering in. So please jump in at any of the four pillars that interest you and start applying these principals.

I am not a doctor or a psychologist, but I know what worked for me, and I believe it will work for you. In my dreams, I see men all over the world rebuilding their health and accomplishing their missions. My sincere intention is that you embrace the four pillars and find the fountain of youth.

Live long and prosper!

Dave Skattum

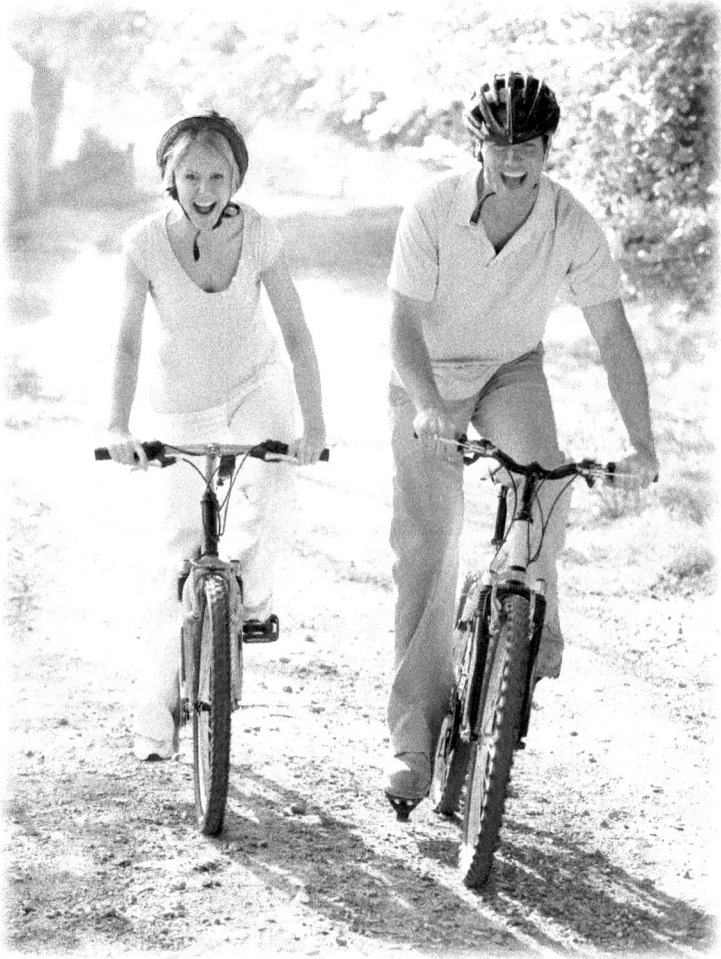

Men's Health

Chapter 1

MEN'S HEALTH—
Finding the Fountain of Youth

*You dream. You plan. You reach.
There will be obstacles. There will be doubters.
There will be mistakes. But with hard work,
with belief, with confidence and trust in yourself
and those around you, there are no limits.*

—Michael Phelps,
23-time Olympic gold medalist swimmer

When I was 49 years old, a friend and colleague was lying in a hospital bed with the doctor leaning over him, sawing his leg off due to diabetic neuropathy. Shortly after that, two more of my friends were diagnosed with diabetes. It almost made my head explode! I thought I was heading in that same direction. I was obese, had a sedentary lifestyle, and ate like a pig.

In the movies, John Wayne and James Bond don't worry about their health. They get shot, beaten and smashed—then get up and finish off the bad guys. Reality, however, is quite different.

John Wayne developed heart disease and had a cancerous lung removed. Ian Fleming, who created James Bond, died from complications of a chest cold because he bucked his doctor's orders and played golf instead.

Look at any health statistics and the real story is the same: men live much shorter lives than women and have higher risks for all 15 leading causes of death except Alzheimer's disease. Despite these statistics, most American men think their health is "excellent"—and they're dying to prove it. Although their health risks are largely preventable, men's infrequent health care—combined with behavior that's better left to Hollywood stuntmen, shortens their lives by more than five years. [MensHealth.org/code/why.html]

What do we men need to do? Where do we begin? For me it began with my friend lying in that hospital bed and then having visions of myself living a miserable, unhealthy life. So, I slowly began to change things in my life: the way I thought, ate and worked out—and I paid more attention to my spiritual life. Today I am running the Ironman triathlon, have lost 75 lbs., have highly nutritious eating habits, and I enjoy a balanced family life and rich spiritual life, all of which has propelled me to share what I've learned and gained with you.

In this book, I want to invite you to come along with me on a journey to much better health and wellness, so you can live your dreams to their fullest. We will focus on four critical areas for extreme health improvement: 1) Changing our thinking, 2) Eating nutritious foods that produce health, 3) Getting our bodies in shape, and 4) Jumping into a deeper spiritual life.

Changing Your Thinking

Your thoughts are creative and powerful. With the right thoughts, you create the right beliefs and you achieve much of what you want. I am a living example of how using correct thinking works. Although I am naturally an optimistic person, as I have matured I realize just how much my thoughts have created my life—the good the bad and the ugly. In Chapter 7 of this book, you will join me in my discovery of the power of those words.

Your thoughts can create a wonderful life, bring you more wealth, more confidence, more success, better relationships—just about anything you want.

However, your thoughts can also make your life miserable, lead to financial disaster, create unneeded struggle, increased emotional pain and more hardships, and force you into dysfunctional relationships—the kind that just don't work or leave you unhappy and unfulfilled. In Chapter 7, we will be talking about purposefully choosing positive and accurate thoughts and how that will change your life.

We will be exploring how affirmations, choosing positive thoughts, and always learning new things will dramatically change your life. And in Chapter 8, we will jump into what happens when we continually strive to grow and improve by learning new things.

Eating Nutritious Foods That Produce Health

I grew up on and live on a ranch in Montana. Hard work and a steady diet of meat and potatoes are a way of life! It took me years of study, experimentation, and some family scorn to realize how important a plant-based diet was for my health. Your food choices each day affect your health and will determine how you feel today, tomorrow and in the future.

Good nutrition is an important part of leading a healthy lifestyle. Combined with physical activity, your diet can help you to reach and maintain a healthy weight, reduce your risk of chronic diseases (like heart disease and cancer) and promote your overall health. Chapter 10 takes an in-depth look at six superfoods that you should strive to eat every day. They can best be remembered with the acronym GBOMBS, which stands for: Greens, Beans, Onions (and Garlic), Mushrooms, Berries, Seeds (and Nuts). We will discuss the amazing impact these six foods will have on your life when you start to eat them every day.

The Standard American Diet—appropriately called the SAD diet—consists mainly of meat, dairy, fat and sugar, as well as refined, processed, and junk foods. Switching to a plant-based diet, shifting to an emphasis on fresh vegetables and fruits, can help prevent and even reverse some of the top killer diseases in the Western world and can even be more effective than medication and surgery. Even after years of eating the SAD diet, it's possible to reduce your risk of degenerative diseases by eating healthier. Toxic hunger and emotional eating are major contributors to poor health and will be discussed in-depth in Chapter 12.

In Chapter 9, I will tell you about my miserable failures with dieting and why typical diets don't work. We will be changing our attitudes about nutrition and in Chapter 11, you will learn about the ANDI Food Scoring system that will help you evaluate the best foods to eat.

Getting Your Body in Shape

You woke up today, you looked in the mirror and you said to yourself, "Gosh darnit! or #%&@)*%$!!—I'm going to get in shape!"

Just one problem—you don't quite know HOW.

It's okay. We've all been there. This might be the first, tenth or fiftieth time you've resolved to get into shape. Sure, things didn't work last time, or the time before that, or even the time before that, but things are going to be different THIS time, right? Never give up that ship!

Here's some good reasons, I think you will agree with me, to get into shape:

- You will have increased self-confidence
- You will get more attention from women
- You will get more respect from men
- You'll become a role model for others
- You will have increased energy and happiness
- Clothes will fit you better
- You will look better naked

- You will sleep better
- You will lower your risk for all types of diseases
- Your self-discipline will spill over to other areas of your life

What does it mean to be in shape? How do you do it? Why should you care? You will learn about three things that will help tremendously to get your body in shape and stay in shape:

1) **Getting started**—Know how and why to get in shape. Find out what works best for you.

2) **Making exercise a lifestyle**—Incorporate your workouts and other healthy habits as a natural part of your life. You wouldn't have it any other way!

3) **Your amazing body**—Appreciate your body as a self-healing, disease-fighting, strong machine!

Jumping into a Deeper Spiritual Life

While I did save spiritual health for last, for me it is the underlying thread that ties my life together. According to a study in Gallup News, statistics show that 95% of us believe in God or a higher power, so I know this is a big deal to many of us. My spiritual life gives me inner strength during hard times. It gives me peace in times of stress and turmoil, and nourishes me with an abiding hope for the future. If I had to choose the most important area to develop in my life, spirituality would be an easy first choice for me.

While it's easy to see the effects of taking care of our physical health through workouts, nutrition and accurate thinking, keeping our spiritual health in check requires a different type of exercise—an internal, soul-searching one. That might seem intimidating, but defining your spirituality doesn't have to be as rigid as a diet. You might want to ask yourself what difference spiritual health has made in the lives of those around you, and if the journey within is worth taking that first step. Just because your spiritual health isn't something you can see in the mirror, doesn't mean that it won't make all the difference in the world—even if it's only in *your* world.

Here are some questions to ask yourself, the answers to which can indicate that you are in good spiritual health:

- Do you have a strong purpose in life?
- Do you have the ability to spend reflective time alone?
- Do you take time to reflect on the meaning of events in life?
- Do you have a clear sense of right and wrong— do you act accordingly?
- Do you have the ability to explain why you believe what you believe?
- Do you care and act for the welfare of others and the environment?
- Are you able to practice forgiveness and compassion toward others?

In future chapters, we will discuss three areas that have helped me grow spiritually. These are prayer, meditation, and fasting. ☑

2

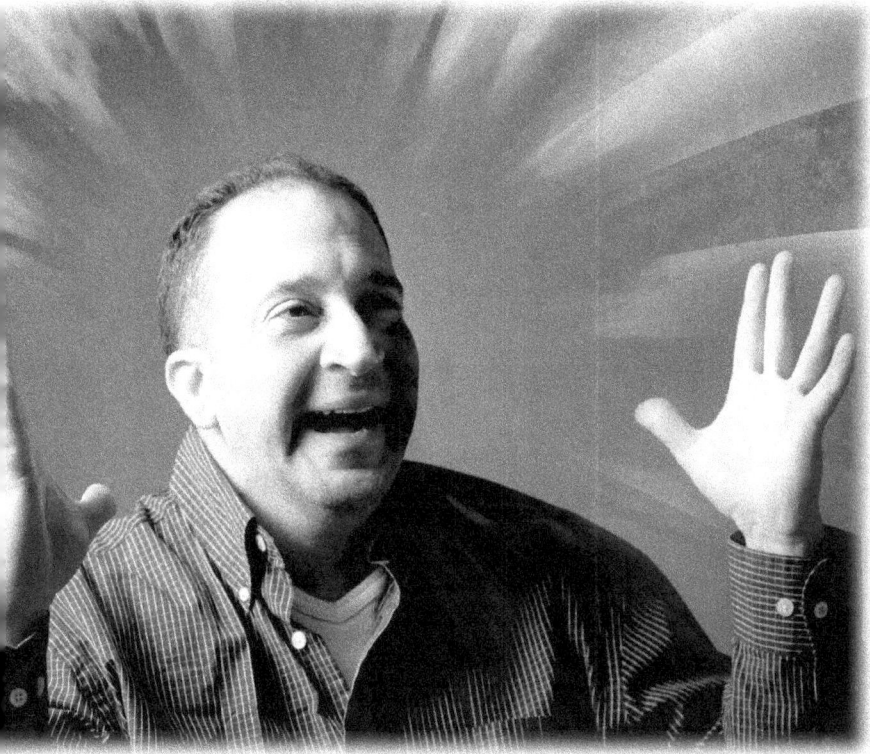

You Are Important

Chapter 2

YOU ARE IMPORTANT—
Be the Rock Star You Are Meant to Be!

Be the reason someone smiles.
Be the reason someone feels loved
and believes in the goodness in people.

—Roy T. Bennett,
The Light in the Heart

Understanding our place in society is foundational to help us get to a healthy place. If each of us realized how truly valuable we are to our family, friends, society and to our Creator, many of our struggles with health would evaporate.

Knowing that our friends and family have love and gratitude for us, and we for them, would replace those nagging negative self-thoughts that drag us into darkness with positive, life-giving thoughts about ourselves and those around us. The tendency to gain weight from emotional eating would be replaced with a sense of mutual respect and appreciation from those around us. The tendency to put off exercise would be replaced with an excited attitude of looking forward to keeping our body fit so we can see our dreams come true and live a long, healthy life with our loved ones. Knowing the important place we have in our world makes it easier to get the physical exercise our bodies need to stay healthy.

In our society, it's sometimes easy for us to think that no one cares about us. So many of us feel alone in a crowd— but there's no need to feel that way! Many of us deal with difficult relationship issues, but even when it seems like we have no support from the people around us, that can be built up.

Besides, the most important thing for us to remember is that God cares about us! He wants us to accept His friendship. He sent His Son so that we might be forgiven. (More on that coming up in later chapters.)

Here are some things to focus on and maybe add to your affirmation list regarding how important you are:

I am important to God because He created me in His image!

The sacred text teaches: *So God created man in His own image; in the image of God He created him; male and female He created them.* [Genesis 1:27] and, *What is man that You are mindful of him, And the son of man that You visit him? For You have made him a little lower than the angels, And You have crowned him with glory and honor.* [Psalms 8:4-5]

Sometimes I just sit and think about this thought—God created us in His image—what a powerful thought! And what are the implications? Take some time and process this on your own.

I matter because I am the only person who can be ME!

Everyone's path in life leads in different directions and we all have a different story to tell. We all face different challenges. We all must learn from different experiences. There are billions of people on this planet and yet YOU are the only person who is exactly like YOU. This simple fact of our unique identity before God is incredibly important. Don't even for a second allow yourself to think anything different.

I am important because I have a special purpose!

No matter who you are, you can provide value. We each have an individual purpose that cannot be compared to everyone else. You have a different perspective to share. Every

11

day, you are guided to shed light on situations that no one else can possibly provide. You can utilize your unique experiences to help and positively influence others.

You have a unique mission in this life! Only you can do it. If you live your life well and seek your highest calling, you will change your world. If you don't or can't because of poor health, it will have a grave effect on the people in your life. So get healthy and stay healthy! You have a lot to do and people around you are depending on you.

I matter because I can help and inspire others!

One of the greatest joys in life is helping and inspiring others along the way and, in turn, being helped and inspired by them, too. We all need support from others—it's human nature. Sometimes, all we need to make our day is for someone to believe in us, and to tell us how much they value and support us.

You can be the one to support others. You can be the one to give someone a positive lift and a helping hand. Helping others not only provides inspiration, but it will also ignite a spark within you. Even when it is not outwardly acknowledged, there is always a return current of energy when we give of ourselves and help others. It's like a continuous circle—when you inspire, you also feel inspired.

I am important because I can turn my life struggles into life lessons!

The old saying goes, "When you are handed lemons, make lemonade!" Life is often challenging; some days are tougher than others. But with every challenge, we gain the opportunity to grow stronger. It's not what life gives us that matters—it's how we deal with the things that life gives. We can continuously improve who we are and what we can achieve, and there's always room for improvement in the way we react when something negative comes our way. Instead of allowing a challenge to bring you down, keep pushing forward, stay cool, and be on the lookout for opportunities. Turn each challenge into a lesson. Others will learn from and be inspired by how you handle things.

I matter because I can love and be loved!

You already know this—loving and receiving love is the ultimate human experience. It's what gives meaning to life. Loving and caring is what adds value to our lives. It provides depth and a reason for living. It provides hope, wonder and excitement. This loving exchange with our partners, kids, friends, and even our pets, is what makes each day worth every challenge and every experience. Remember that there is no greater love than what we can share with our Creator— and no earthly love can compare.

I am important because I can provide joy and happiness!

You know the joy you get when you provide happiness to another person. Take time to tell those around you how much you do care. It helps you as much as it helps them. Give them a high five, a hug or a smile. And don't stop at just telling them; SHOW THEM each day with acts of kindness. Spread your cheer and good humor everywhere you go. Why hide it under a bushel basket? [Matthew 5:15-16] You never know whose day you may brighten up.

My friend Rob owns a construction business. One of his employees decided to build himself a house in his off hours, a major undertaking. Rob could see that he was struggling and overwhelmed. So, one weekend when Rob knew his friend was out of town he took his whole crew down and framed in the whole subfloor on this guy's new house.

The employee came back on Sunday night and was overwhelmed with gratitude, filled with joy and happiness—a gift that guy will never forget. Way to go, Rob!

I matter because I can show others that anything is possible!

The passion and determination to become a healthy person will take you farther than you can imagine. If you just settle, or are afraid to take chances, you will not reach that true-life potential. Let go of fear; take chances and do your best. There is a saying that, "If you aim at nothing, you'll hit the mark every time." Set goals. Take each day step-by-step, but also write down your long-term goals and log your progress and growth. Determination, passion, and the willingness to keep moving forward consistently are the true keys to long-term success. See Chapter 3 for a deeper look at taking the next steps.

I am important because I can influence others to achieve their own greatness!

Be a leader. Leadership is about inspiring and influencing others to achieve their own greatness. No matter who you are, you can positively influence and lead others. You can lend a helping hand, and encourage others. You can make a difference in their lives. Never underestimate yourself or your capabilities. Be passionate. Be genuine. Be yourself. And always remember that you matter—you are important.

I am a member of Toastmasters International, an organization with the goal of helping people improve their communication and leadership skills. The highest personal level a person can achieve is to become a Distinguished Toastmaster. It's quite an honor and involves a lot of hard work in the areas of personal and leadership development.

Being a driven person, I set my eyes on that goal and achieved it—not once but four times. (My wife tells me I am all-or-nothing. I have no idea what's she talking about!)

Since then, several of my Toastmasters friends have also applied themselves and received this distinction. I can't help but think I had a little to do with inspiring them. You too can inspire others around you to do something amazing. What will it be?

I matter because God sent Jesus Christ to Earth to help me find my way through this life and into the next!

This is my experience and the sacred text explains it well: "This is how much God loved the world: He gave his Son, His one and only Son. And this is why: so that no one need be destroyed; by believing in Him, anyone can have a whole and lasting life." [John 3:16] How can you go wrong knowing such a thing? The Creator of the universe loves you completely.

Once we truly know in our hearts how important we are to God and to each other, we will have the foundation upon which great health in body, mind and spirit can be attained. ☑

3

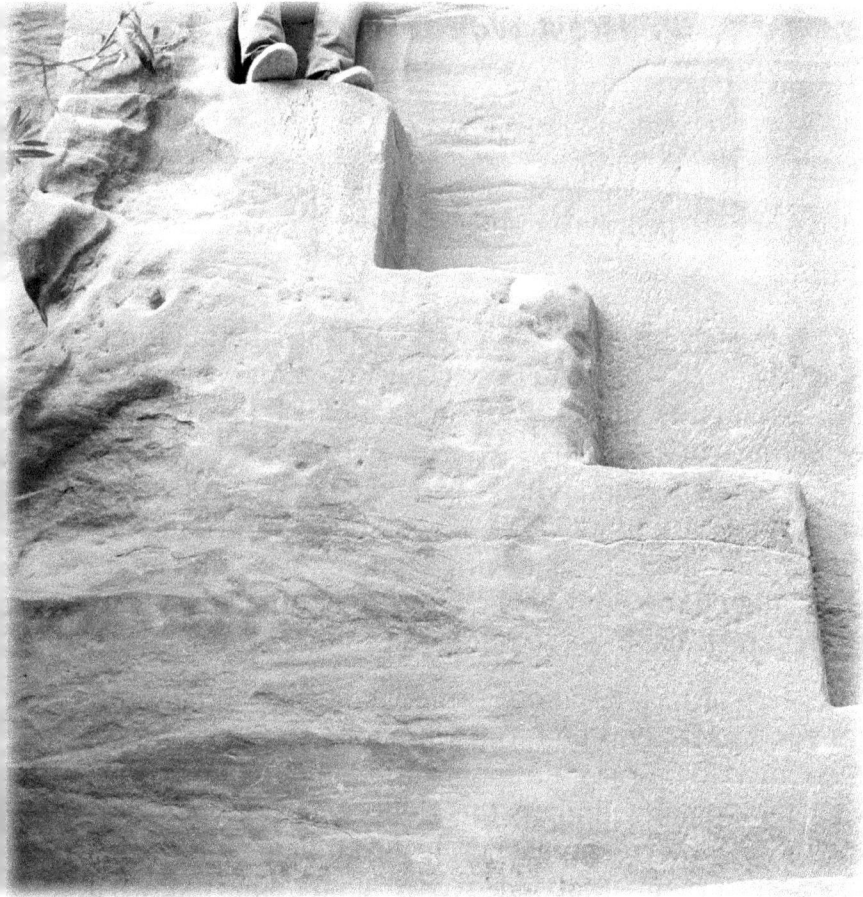

Baby Steps

CHAPTER 3

BABY STEPS—
Fastest Way to the Top!

Life's a marathon,
not a sprint.

—Dr. Phillip McGraw, American television
personality, author and psychologist

Recently my son Josh and I did a 28-mile trail run in our beloved Absaroka Beartooth Mountains. There's something awe inspiring about being high up in the rugged wilderness that sets my soul free. But it wasn't too long ago for me that such an endeavor could be only a dream. In fact, I remember a short hike I took with my son and daughter that nearly did me in. I was having so much back and knee pain that I didn't know if I was going to get home. How did I go from barely-making-it to ultra-trail-runner? BABY STEPS.

I had to take about three years of gradually running longer and faster. I had to learn about nutrition and how to feed my body for such a long run. I learned about using the right equipment, finding the right shoes, proper clothing, hydration packs, compact survival gear, and predator protection. Any monumental endeavor in life requires that we break it down into manageable steps, setting measurable goals, and keeping at it.

This process will be required for all of us as we begin to get healthier. Nutrition, exercise, good thinking, and spirituality all require that we start where we're at, and begin to take small steps toward achieving great health.

I tend to get in a hurry, to overcommit, and then to get discouraged, forgetting that the journey is usually more rewarding than the destination. The pace of life has increased. Rushing through our days—our lives—has now become the norm. We want everything now: happiness now, success now, health now, love now! Not surprisingly, this is the way many of us approach our goals and life changes as well. Patience is hard to come by. If we haven't reached our goal yesterday, it must be because we're not working hard enough or fast enough, or we're lazy and undisciplined.

Hard work and discipline are certainly valuable traits when trying to make changes in our lives or attain important goals; however, even diligence and persistence are often not enough to get the results we're looking for. The lack of an effective strategy (breaking it down into baby steps) is often our greatest obstacle. In our impatience for results, we try to change too much at once and expect too much of ourselves. This impatience usually leads to frustration and failure.

Sometimes we don't even take the first step because our dreams, goals, and desires seem so overwhelming, so intimidating, and so unachievable that we give up before we even start.

Maybe we just need to try a different strategy. Dr. Phil says, "Life is a marathon, not a sprint." That same philosophy can be applied when we're attempting to make life changes, whether it's in career advancement, building a business, educational, weight-loss or fitness goals, eating right, thinking right, or getting right with God.

Learn to Take Baby Steps

This may be the simplest, yet the most effective strategy we can use, because consistency and learning to build on small victories are the keys to success. The happiest and most successful people will tell you that they have achieved everything by taking small steps and making one positive choice after another.

Start Looking for the Mini-Victories

What's a mini-victory? It's a completion of a baby step—a realistic, quickly achievable, small portion of a larger objective. Baby steps will vary depending upon our specific intention, timeframe and motivation. The reason this strategy works is because we can see tangible progress rather quickly, so we feel a sense of accomplishment and are encouraged to move on to our next mini-goal. We then use the small successes as stepping-stones to larger change. Here are a couple of examples:

Consider Nutritional Goals

When we are attempting to eat better food, don't expect to go from eating Big Macs, french fries and a coke, to salads, soups and smoothies overnight. You will doom yourself to failure. Try adding a delicious fruit smoothie to your breakfast for a few weeks. Once you've made that a habit, start adding kale (what's that?) to the smoothie, then carrots, then broccoli. Over time, you'll find yourself desiring this type of food even more. Swap out one unhealthy snack for a piece of fruit, or eat one vegetarian meal a week, and replace one soda or cappuccino with a glass of water. When we try to eliminate all sugar or soda or junk food from our diets cold-turkey, we usually fall off the wagon within the first week or two.

Consider Exercise Goals

Train to run a 5K, then a 10K, then a half-marathon rather than training for the full marathon all at once. This advice holds true even when tackling the full marathon. Many successful long-distance runners say that they don't run 26 miles—they run 1 mile, 26 times.

Most of us want career success, but it usually comes one rung up the ladder at a time. Take one course at a time. Achieve one certification. Improve one skill.

This strategy is useful in almost every area of life and when trying to achieve nearly any goal. Just take baby steps, work towards one mini-victory at a time, and make sure you celebrate each achievement in some small way—*no, not with that donut!* A little success goes a long way in propelling you to the finish line.

Why Taking Baby Steps Is the Best Path to Great Health

When we watch TV or browse the Internet, our inquiries into how to improve our health and happiness are often met with an endless supply of quick-fixes like diets, meditation videos, the latest fad product or fitness workout. In the craziness of our lives, we don't think we have the time for much else so we find a diet or cleanse that makes the most attractive promises and we do the workout plans that are short, quick, intense, and that make the most attractive promises.

If we don't see remarkable results quickly—if we don't sweat our butts off during a workout or "sweat it" through a 10-day lemon-cayenne cleanse—it doesn't seem worth it, so we give up on it. No pain, no gain, right? We are often sold the idea that positive life changes can come from drastic action in a super-short amount of time and it's exciting to think this, because who wouldn't want it as fast as possible? There's only one hitch: the "results" from these quick fixes don't last either, and they don't make us healthier or happier in the long run.

I love getting out on my road bike (pedaling that is) and riding the roads around my house in our beautiful valley that is nestled on the western edge of the Absaroka-Beartooth Wilderness. There's something about the views and the wind blowing through my hair that is energizing. My favorite loop is about 17 miles long. When I first started, I remember taking two snack breaks before I got home. It took me about two hours. After a couple of years of riding and improving my equipment, I got that down to about an hour. My fastest time was an 18-mph average.

That was quite an improvement, right? But I wanted a little more speed. Maybe I could reach a 22-mph average? I worked hard for quite a while but seemed to hit a plateau. While surfing the web I came across an ad that read: "Do you want to improve your bike speed? Guaranteed 15% speed improvement in only 90 days!" What was I to do? It was only $159! Out came the credit card and I jumped into it. After 90 days, I hadn't improved much. At the end of the 90 days, I celebrated with a bike crash and ended up dislocating my shoulder. Lesson learned for me: it's better to take baby steps and enjoy the journey!

What Can We Do to Live Healthier and Happier in Today's World?

We need to move beyond the "no pain, no gain" idea and instead consider this: No pain, all gain! One can achieve true, sustained health and happiness by taking small, continuous, and most importantly, gentle steps forward—the very opposite of a quick-fix paradigm. Incrementally add things into our life (healthy foods, exercise, accurate thinking and spiritual health) in amounts that don't add large amounts of stress to our already stressful life, and only what can be reasonably sustained. Increase and move on to the next step when we're ready.

This approach enhances the quality of our lives—it begins an actual transition to increased health and happiness. It immediately shows us what diets and workout plans cannot: what it feels like to be a person who treats himself well and deserves to be treated well. This approach reminds us that what we truly want is what we *think* weight loss (or ripped abs) can deliver for us: to feel good in our bodies, and happier in our lives.

By easing our way in with small steps, we come to understand that health and happiness is a long-term pursuit and involves a much bigger picture than anything a quick-fix can deliver. The simple fact is that yo-yo dieting and unsustainable workout plans add stress to our bodies and minds, while small improvements change our lives over time with minimal or no added stress.

We are a natural species living in an unnatural world. The concept of quick-fixes is as foreign to our natural design as is the idea of "no pain, no gain." (There are no diets, workout schedules, or calorie counting in nature.) Our bodies are designed to do the very best they can every minute of every day to stay alive. When we minimize self-inflicted pain, only then do we see what real gains look like.

Being a healthy man takes desire and consistent effort, requires change, and is not automatic. One of the tools each of us should have in our mental toolbox is the concept of BABY STEPS. Success comes when we take a first step towards good health, enjoy the feeling when we succeed, then repeat. ☑

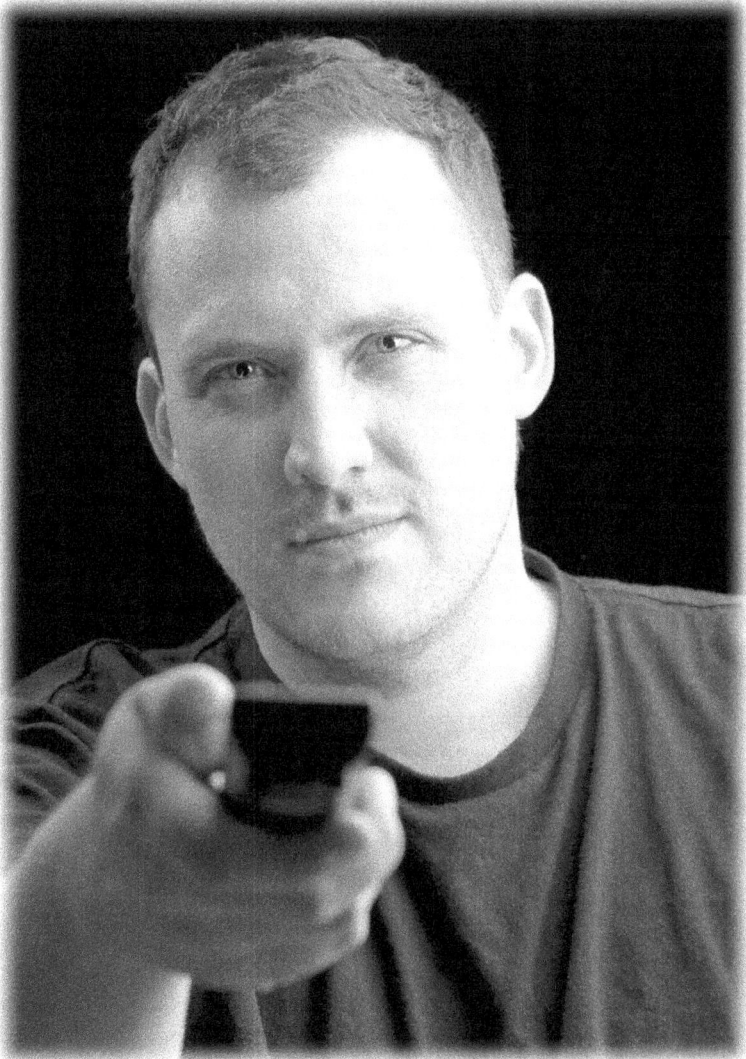

4

Creating a New You

CHAPTER 4

CREATING A NEW YOU—
Doing What It Takes
to Bring On Real Change

As you shake off the old way of being,
the false self that society caused to you create,
you get to discover yourself anew—
only this self is your authentic self,
your true self.

—Barra, *Awakening to the Truth of Self*

The human body has incredible machinery for regenerating itself and creating a new you. Your outer layer of skin, the epidermis (there are 24 layers in all), replaces itself every 35 days. You are given a new liver every six weeks (a human liver can regenerate itself completely even if as little as 25% of it remains). Your stomach lining replaces itself every 4 days, and the stomach cells that come into contact with digesting food are replaced every 5 minutes! Our entire skeletal structure is regenerated every 3 months. Your entire brain replaces itself every two months. And the entire human body, right down to the last atom, is replaced every 5-to-7 years.

Good nutrition plays a key role in how effective your body is at replacing and repairing itself. (See Chapter 11 for a list of excellent foods to consume for best results.) The better the food you eat, the healthier your new body will become.

Our bodies are in a constant state of change and growth—it's automatic and built in to the design. But what about your current situation? Are you where you want to be with your health and fitness? Are you where you want to be with great nutrition, healthy thinking, and an active spirituality? If you're like me, there are many areas in your life that can use some positive change. Unlike your body, this kind of change takes effort, determination and planning. And yet, once you get started, you'll find that all areas of your life will thrive (in a built-in, automatic way) once great habits are well established. Here are ten steps I use to create lasting change in my life:

1) Have laser-focused belief.

You need to have a firm belief, without any doubt, in the achievement and success of your desires. These beliefs need to be like unquestioned commands communicated directly into your subconscious mind. They will shape every thought, feeling and action you'll take. Within the strength of these beliefs lies the "core" to real and everlasting change. When I was jolted to reality by my friend having his leg amputated because of diabetes and years of poor lifestyle choices, I decided I had to change before my poor choices got the best of me. I became consumed with the belief that I could get healthy—and I have.

2) Keep your beliefs managed and under control.

If not, no matter what you decide to change, you'll never have the wherewithal and conviction to achieve your goals or the sufficient wattage behind your desire to truly change. If you have a monumental dream (and you should!), you will have to break it down into manageable steps and then take it one step at a time.

3) Create a vision and a strategy.

Imagine yourself having completed your goals. How do you look? How do you feel about yourself? What are others saying about you? What does health, fitness, great vigor and vitality, and success look like to you? Write these things down, in the present tense, starting with the words, "I am now..." This becomes your vision statement.

Next, determine and write down what must happen for you to know that you've made the desired changes in your life. What would be the final step or results achieved? Would it be that you could run a certain distance at a certain pace? Would it be that people comment on the new you? Now you've got measurable goals to focus on, include specific and descriptive words—use emotional word pictures that describe how you now feel. Include some steps on how you will get there. This becomes your mission statement.

I recently used a 3-step development process for a project I am working on called Run723.com. As I walked through this process, it really helped me describe what I wanted it to be, what I wanted it to do, and what kind of an organization it would be.

First came the **Mission**. It describes what I want Run723.com to do. "We will run every trail in the Absaroka-Beartooth Wilderness and provide a platform for discovering and enjoying the wilderness through a blog site. We also want to provide tools and resources to help others enjoy the Absaroka-Beartooth Wilderness."

Second was the **Vision**. This describes what it will look like in the future. "We will bring the majesty of the Absaroka-Beartooth Wilderness to the masses and inspire others to join the running (or hiking) challenge and experience this wilderness."

Third was coming up with our **Core Values**. Who we are as a group. "We are inclusive, prepared, generous, adventurous, and we care for the wilderness."

Going through this three-step process helped me encapsulate what Run723.com will be about. If you go through this same process on any project you are planning, you will be much closer to the place you're heading. With your

Mission, Vision and Core Values in place, you will be able to say *yes* to things you should do, and *no* to things you shouldn't do.

4) Choose the steps you will take.

Write down several steps you can take each day that will assist you on your journey toward the new you. This is no small part of the process. It will allow these new patterns to be ingrained into your subconscious mind and ultimately enable you to create new habits. In the areas of exercise and nutrition, for example, your steps might include:

- Set the alarm clock 45 minutes early.

- Have workout clothes laid out the night before for easy accessibility.

- Take the dog on your walk—you'll have companionship and the dog will benefit from the exercise, too.

- Have a healthy lunch prepared the night before.

- Stock your fridge with healthy snacks you can grab quickly when you're hungry.

- Plan all your meals in advance.

- Schedule exercise, meals, and other healthy activities into your day planner or smartphone.

5) Be specific and have measurable goals.

Write down a date when you'll start these new strategies and how often you'll do them. Choose the route you'll take in the neighborhood for your run, or which gym you'll visit. State exactly in the present tense what you're doing, as in, "I am walking three miles today. I will do so on Monday, Wednesday and Friday each week." This is much better than simply saying, "I will exercise each week." Being specific implies a commitment to your goals and makes them easier to measure.

6) Make a commitment to start.

Think about what's at stake and focus again on the list you made, thinking about how it'll feel and what benefits you'll receive when you incorporate this strategic change into your life. We've all had the experience of wanting to start an exercise program "next week"; when next week comes and goes, we just put things off, and it never happens. Make the commitment to begin—and follow through.

I struggle with committing to a weightlifting program. I know it will have a dramatic effect on my physical performance and health if I can build up some muscle mass. But every time I try it I only last a few weeks. Today I found a *Bowflex* on Craigslist for $100—I'll keep you posted.

Motivation can come from both fear of loss AND from anticipation of gain. I have a gutter business along with my son Josh (see GutterMontana.biz). In our advertising, we often use "pain shots" such as clogged gutters and people falling off roofs—it works! Personally, I will never forget the sound of that power saw amputating my friend's leg! In the programs we're starting here, your very life and health are truly at stake, so if fearing the worst works for you, then use it to your advantage. AND remember that anticipating the great benefits and rewards is an even BETTER motivator. Just ask Pavlov's dogs!

7) Thank yourself—and God—for participating!

Celebrate your success! It's OK to be grateful to yourself. This is a wonderful affirmation. Hearing the words "thank you" relaxes the muscles (even the DNA) and deepens your resolve. If someone thanks you for something, it naturally makes you feel good. You want to keep doing it to get that praise again—so praise and thank yourself often. Soon others will see the positive changes in your life and start praising you, too.

There are common themes in Christian circles that all the praise and glory goes to God, and that without the strength of the Savior, we could accomplish nothing. I believe this is true and I do send praise and gratitude back to the source of all that is good for my every accomplishment. I recommend this because, when you do it, there is a feedback loop of positive energy (the returning of your love and gratitude from the Creator and his Son multiplied), that far exceeds the "horizontal feedback" you'll get from friends and associates.

8) Notice it when you don't follow through.

Ask yourself why, but be careful not to beat up yourself over a relapse. Do you need to alter the motivation or the steps to your new strategy? Was there something that created some doubt in your mind? If so, change it back. The results you get are the product of your thinking, so if you continue to be disappointed at what you achieve, you must be willing to ask yourself some hard questions and change your beliefs.

At the core of many self-improvement modalities (in AA, for sure) are the concepts of triggers and the moment of decision. It's always good to self-examine when you experience a setback. What happened that triggered that downward turn? Did someone criticize or upset you because of a mistake that either you or they made? Did that trigger a need for an old form of self-gratification? A bad habit that you're almost, but not quite, over with? There's a moment of decision in there—it's often ignored, but it's always there anyway. Being more self-aware before you take the leap will lead to more moments of right decision.

9) Use your affirmations.

Often people will take the affirmations they've created and make an audio recording of them that can be played back each morning as they exercise, on the morning commute, etc. This is a great way to start the day on a positive and upbeat note while encouraging yourself to commit to your new habit.

One of my affirmations was, "To enjoy it as my audience stands to a thunderous applause." I joined my local Toastmasters club and this has actually happened to me. They work!

10) Keep a journal of your progress.

Did you ever go to the gym and use a personal trainer to get started? Remember how they have a chart to log every exercise you do by the week, and you get to watch the pounds you're lifting go up and up? Remember how satisfying that was to watch your progress? Do that for everything! This is very important.

Journaling is a way to keep track of how far you've come and how much you've accomplished, which can sometimes be difficult for you to remember. Journaling can be as simple as a brief paragraph noting what days you performed a certain habit or task and what the outcome was. You can also use a journal to record specifics of your diet and exercise regime as well as how you're feeling as a whole, and any emotional and even spiritual events that are occurring. It's important to do this daily. The more specific you are with your journaling, the better reference tool it will become. Who knows? Maybe someday I'll be reading YOUR book!

Creating a new you is happening on the inside whether you are participating or not. Now is the time to be proactive. Set your sights high. Take charge of your life and create the YOU that you want and that you KNOW you can become! ☑

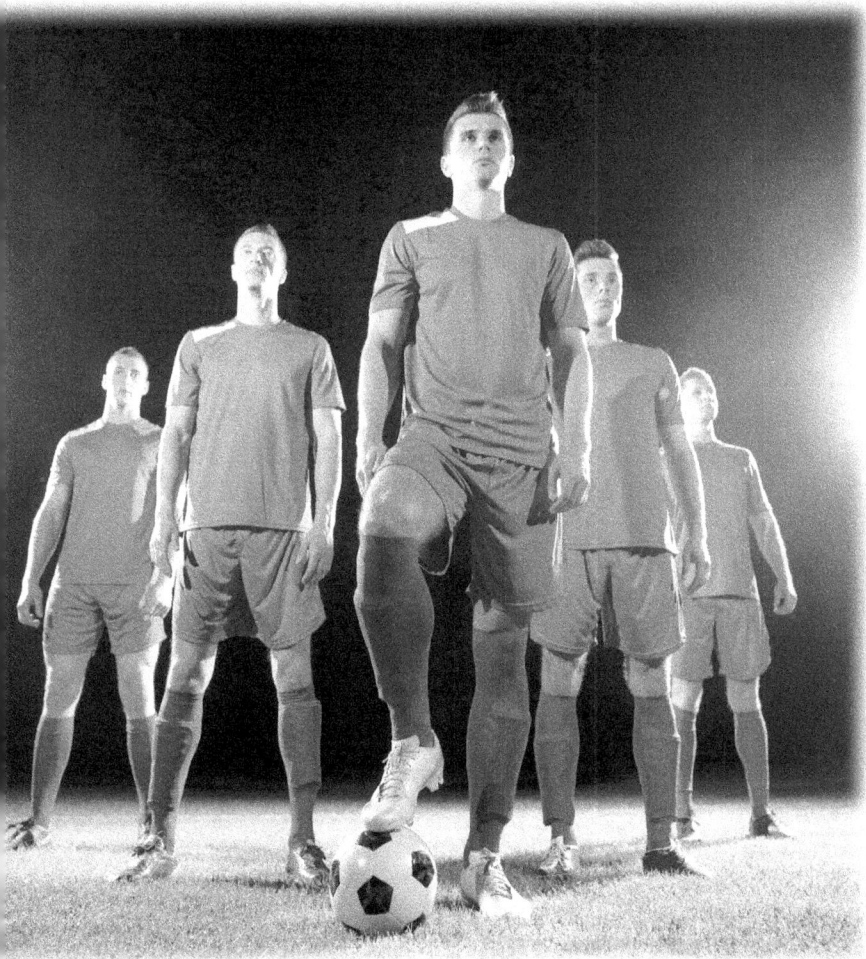

5

Build a Team

CHAPTER 5

BUILD A TEAM—
Get Support to Change Your Life

*Talent wins games, but teamwork
and intelligence wins championships.*

—Michael Jordan

In my twenties, I started a business. I had high hopes and I just knew things were going to be amazing—I would make a bunch of money, have tons of people working with me and I would be happy. Well, it didn't happen the way I planned. The business was at best semi-successful and I did make some money and at times I did have a bunch of people working with me. But the truth is it never was what I had hoped for. Looking back on those years I think the biggest mistake I made was not asking for help and advice. Having a team of smart people around me could have saved me so much grief and expense.

It is the same way with our health. We need people who are experts in areas we are not. We need people around us who can motivate us when we are down. We need trusted people around us when we require a kick in the pants.

To get healthy we should build a team of people around us to help us. Here are some ideas for team members:

Your Doctor

Doctors can help you proceed in a healthy manner and pace. They can talk to you about your individual needs and give you ideas. I recommend that you see your family doctor annually, but there's no one-size-fits-all answer, says Heidi Doyle, PA-C, a physician assistant with Duke Primary Care

North Hills. "Regular check-ups are important to maintain a relationship with your doctor and to receive individualized counseling based on your family health history and your lifestyle. Age and disease risk are the primary factors influencing when to get a physical," says Doyle.

Here's what you need to know: If you're under 30 and healthy—don't smoke, no disease risk factors (including being overweight) and don't take prescription medications-get a check-up every two to three years. If you are age 30–40, healthy individuals should get a physical every other year. Annual physicals start around age 50. That's also when men should undergo colonoscopies to screen for colon cancer. Repeat every 10 years unless there is a family history of colon cancer, colon polyps, or the test results are abnormal. Different recommendations about check-up frequency apply to individuals who take medication and have chronic disease risk factors. In that case, annual physicals may be recommended since blood tests may be necessary and treatments may need to be changed.

Being overweight also influences how often you get a physical because it increases one's risk for high blood pressure, high cholesterol and diabetes. "For these individuals, the annual physical is an opportunity to reinforce healthy lifestyle choices," Doyle says. "The key is for each person to be responsible for their own health," adds Doyle. "A person with diabetes, high blood pressure or high cholesterol, or one who is simply more susceptible to those conditions, can make lifestyle changes that are much more impactful than any pill I can prescribe."

A Nutritionist

Your physical health is key to your active lifestyle. Like a car, your body won't run without the right fuel. With your new lifestyle, you must take special care to make sure you're taking in enough calories, vitamins and other nutrients to keep you going strong. Having a knowledgeable nutritionist to give you advice about a balanced, nutritional diet will be invaluable.

Listed below are some opening questions on nutrition that you can begin to think about to get you started in the right direction and to discuss with your nutritionist:

How much should I eat?

The amount of food you need varies based on your age, size and activity level. Generally, you need to consume foods that replenish the amount of energy you burn each day. The amount of energy provided by a food is measured in calories. Most people need between 1,500 and 2,000 calories a day. However, for many athletes, this number can increase by as much as 1,000 to 1,500 calories or more. Teen athletes, who need enough fuel for both intense training and rapid growth and development, may need as many as 5,000 calories daily. While everyone's needs are different, you can learn over time how to balance your calorie needs to perform at a high level, and avoid excessive weight loss or gain.

What kind of calories should I eat?

Calories come in different forms, including carbohydrates, fats and proteins:

Carbohydrates are your body's best source of calories. Carbohydrates are found in everything from fruit and veggies to junk food. There are 2 types of carbohydrates: simple and complex. Simple carbohydrates (like yogurt, flour and fruit juice) are easier for your body to break down, so they can give you a rapid burst of energy. Complex carbohydrates (like GBOMBS, see Chapter 10) take longer to break down in the body. They are a better source of energy over time, just as a log burns longer and makes a better source of heat than a piece of paper. The complex carbohydrates found in whole grain products are considered the most beneficial. Examples of complex carbohydrates include whole-grain bread, potatoes, brown rice, oatmeal and kidney beans.

Fat is another important source of calories. In limited amounts, fat is a necessary fuel source and serves other important functions for your health, such as supporting healthy skin and hair. However, too much fat can lead to heart disease and other health problems. Further, replacing carbohydrates in your diet with fat can slow you down, as your body must work harder to use fat for energy. When possible, choose unsaturated fats, such as those found in olive oil and nuts. These fats are better for your heart.

You should limit saturated fats and avoid trans fats altogether. These fats can raise your low-density lipoprotein (LDL) cholesterol levels, which increases your risk of heart disease and type 2 diabetes.

Nutritionists recommend that **protein** make up the remaining 10% to 15% of your daily calories. Protein is found in foods like meat, eggs, milk, beans and nuts.

What nutrients do I need?

You need the same 50 vitamins and minerals as everyone else. To stay healthy, just be sure the extra calories you take in each day are nutrient dense—full of calcium, iron, potassium and other healthy vitamins and minerals. Although it can be tempting to reach for junk food as an easy source of calories, focus instead on lean meats, whole grains and a variety of fruits and vegetables to fuel your body. Dropping GBOMBS every-day gives you a vast array of micro- and macro-nutrients, packed full of needed vitamins and minerals.

What if I want to lose weight?

Your body needs a lot of energy, vitamins and minerals to keep you at optimal performance. Because of this, restrictive diet plans can harm your abilities and damage your health. Without the calories provided by carbohydrates, protein and fat, you may not have the energy and endurance to remain productive. Further, less food often leads to malnutrition. What has worked for me is to follow Dr. Fuhrman's nutrition plan and I also became a Nutritarian. Seek out whole, organic fruits and vegetables, and drop GBOMBS every day. Avoid processed foods and sugars.

Although I don't have a personal nutritionist, I have recently enrolled in a nutrition course with the Nutritarian Educational Institute. It's like having a nutritionist—every time I begin a new segment or read a new chapter, I am learning new things that super-charge my nutrition.

Form a Mastermind Group

Many times, when I have encountered a particularly challenging situation or wanted to start something new in my life, I have started a mastermind group. I call a couple like-minded friends and someone I know who is knowledgeable about the issue I am facing and ask them all to meet with me over a designated period of time to work through the situa-tion. It's amazing the creativity, energy and solutions that come out of a group like that. I have never been disappointed.

For example, a few months ago I came to a block in my life regarding my website. I was frustrated and inexperienced. So, I called up two friends. One was an expert problem solver and the other had a website I liked and she had done it herself. We met five times over the next month. The results were stunning. Not only did I get a great website out of the deal, but I also was able to assist my friends in their endeavors.

Family

Of all the people in the world, some of the most important are your immediate family. Don't forget to include them in your plan. They know you best and have a vested interest in you being healthy. Encourage them to join you on your journey to good health.

Spiritual Advisor

Getting and staying in touch with your inner spiritual person takes a lot of work and effort. It would be time well spent to spend time with a respected spiritual figure. Someone who has "been there and done that" adds so much value to the development of our spiritual lives. I meet with my spiritual advisor almost weekly and every time I come away with a new challenging insight. Keeps me sharp and humble.

Find a Buddy

How important is male bonding and guy time for men? Do we really need to spend time with other guys just to feel good? Evolutionary studies show that men really open up and reveal their true colors only when they're with other men. Guy time among men is often based on shared activities, instead of emotional sharing, which is more typical of women's friendships. Stereotypical common activities of the typical guy time include watching sports on television, working together, or going out for coffee.Men who have close male friends are healthier, happier and more successful.

Massage Therapist

Professional athletes and their coaches have sworn by massage therapy for years, going so far as to keep massage therapists on the payroll indefinitely. Until recently, there hasn't been conclusive evidence that massage really does have a positive effect on athletes.

However, thanks to new studies and some backing by reputable sources, the benefits of massage are being taken seriously. And those benefits are not just for the pros. They're extended to anyone who participates in a regular exercise program.

According to the American Massage Therapy Association (AMTA), massage acts to improve performance, reduce pain, prevent injury, encourage focus and shorten recovery time. It basically involves two types of responses: a mechanical response as a result of the pressure and movement and a reflex response where the nerves respond to the stimulation of a massage.

It's important to note that therapists and research suggest that a massage here and there is nice, but won't give you the same benefits as a regular massage program. Like exercise itself, your benefits are cumulative, meaning the more regularly you receive a massage, the more you'll reap their advantages. Think of it as preventative maintenance. Know that the benefits are often short-lived and part of the reason why it is a cumulative action.

Massage therapist Paul Valentine recommends scheduling "once a week if possible or every other week if you're training at a high level." If getting a weekly or bi-weekly massage isn't in the budget or you don't have time, he suggests aiming for twice a month.

Physical Therapist

If you are active, eventually you will get hurt. This isn't a pessimistic perspective, it's simply an unfortunate reality of repetitive motion. A physical therapist can help your body heal in the fastest way possible. Years ago, I was using a table saw and cut two fingers off and mutilated my thumb. The incredible doctor was able to sew the two fingers back on and do some major reconstructive work on my thumb. I still remember him saying to me, "this will take a while to heal, but if you do what your physical therapist tells you to do you should have very good use of your hand." ...You guessed it. I didn't and to this day I regret not spending more time and effort with that physical therapist.

Chiropractor

Many people swear by the positive effects of chiropractic care when talking about their personal successes. When the spine exhibits imperfections in movement and/or alignment, the resulting vertebral subluxations can create focal areas of irritation in the nervous system, which subsequently interfere with the optimum functions of all other systems. As a result, our performance suffers.

Performance Coach

If you are going for a big goal in your life you might want to consider taking it to a new level by hiring a high-performance coach. They work with an individual to challenge and support him or her in achieving higher levels of performance while allowing them to bring out the best in themselves and those around them. Performance coaching helps the individual align beliefs and actions to create a desired outcome, and build relationships based on honesty and accountability. The reason someone would use a performance coach would be to help them better focus on goals and development for the future.

A high-performance coach can help the client explore alternative ideas, solutions, evaluate options and make decisions. They also challenge client assumptions and perspectives to provoke new ideas, stretch goals, and stimulate action.

I hired a triathlon coach when I was getting into triathlons. He helped me be successful quicker and helped me pace myself in a healthier way.

Don't try to be a lone ranger out there. It doesn't work, trust me!! Build a team of people around you and your life will be healthier, wealthier and wiser! ☑

First Pillar

Accurate Thinking

6

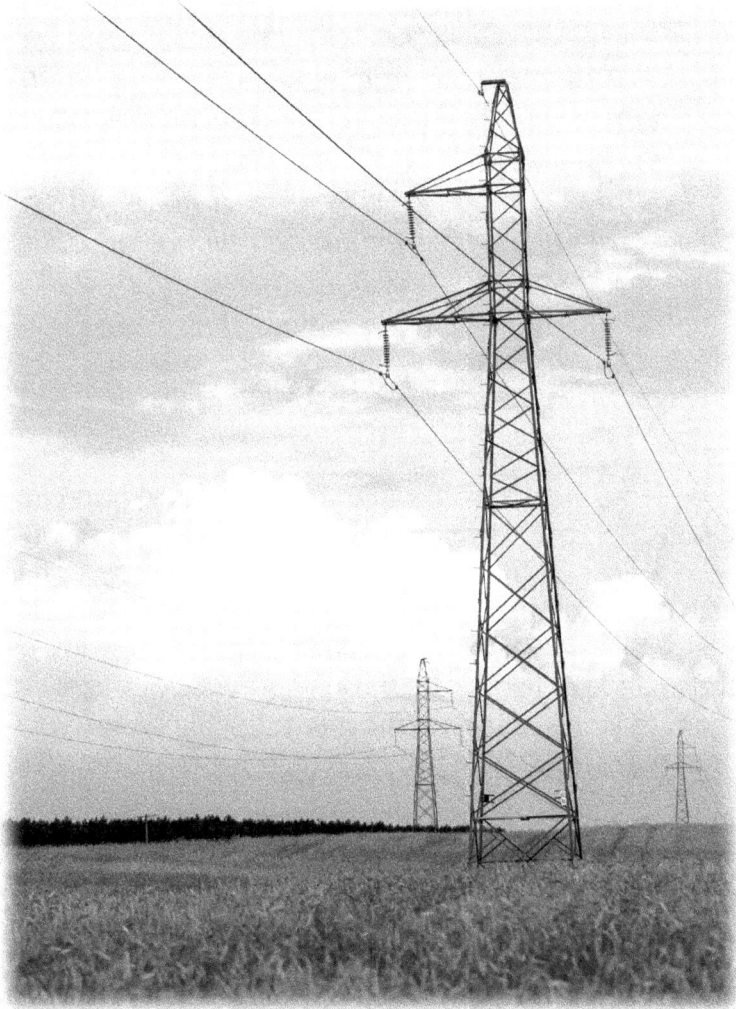

Affirmations

CHAPTER 6

AFFIRMATIONS—
The Power of "I Am"

*A man's mind may be likened to a garden,
which may be intelligently cultivated or allowed
to run wild; but whether cultivated or neglected,
it must, and will, bring forth. If no useful seeds
are put into it, then an abundance of useless
weed seeds will fall therein, and will
continue to produce their kind.*

—James Allen, *As a Man Thinketh*

A business coach once asked me to do an experiment. He said, "Dave, write down ten things you want to accomplish in your life. Then, one-by-one, imagine you have completed them. What have you done? What are you feeling?" Then he advised, "Now, write down each of those accomplishments in one sentence and start repeating them to yourself three time a day. It will change your life."

At first, I thought it was a bunch of B.S., but I was paying the guy to advise me, so I did it. For the first month or so, it felt hypocritical, like I was lying to myself. But then things started to change—I began to change. Today, 7 years later, I have accomplished many of those dreams, some have changed, and some are still in my future. But I believe they have become an important part of what makes me who I am today. To me, affirmations are like prayers—they call the Power of the Universe to my side.

An affirmation is usually a sentence or phrase that you repeat 2–3 times a day to make a declaration to yourself and to the Universe affirming your intention for this to be the truth in your world. We all have in our brains a thing called a Reticular Activating System (RAS), which is like a filter that lets in information that we need and filters out information that we don't. If we didn't have this system, we would be bombarded with so much information that our senses would overload and we would go into massive overwhelm. Instead, our brain registers what matters to us based on our goals, needs, interests, and desires. Keep in mind, as mentioned in our opening quote, that if you don't use this power actively, your subconscious backlog of "weeds"—past fears, failures, traumas, and resentments—will be passively programming the RAS for you, probably creating negative outcomes behind your back!

When you say an affirmation repeatedly, a couple of things happen. One is that it sends a very clear message to your RAS that these concepts are important to you. When you do that, it gets busy noticing ways to help you achieve your goals. If reaching your ideal weight is your emphasis, you will suddenly begin to feel more desire to work out, and nutritious foods will gain in their appeal to you. If more prosperity is your goal, investment and earning opportunities will move to the forefront of your awareness and may even drop into your lap! Your affirmations will kick your creativity into a higher gear. Here are four steps I have used in developing affirmations in my life:

1) Identified Negative Self-Talk and Beliefs

This is a process I am continually working through. It is like a person with a gold detector—the more and deeper I look, the more negative self-talk I discover. The other day, I was talking with a good friend and was telling him about a business that I had started in my past. To me it was old hat—old Dave story stuff. I remembered a lot of the negative events about the business, like the financial struggles, the time away from family, and the poor decisions I made. I was really focused on the negative parts of that part of my life. So, my friend's response shocked me, he said something like, "Dave, that's amazing that you could start a business like that and have some really good success with it. When most people start a business, they fail within a couple of years." I knew I had found another negative story I had been telling myself. Now I tell myself a more accurate story about that experience.

When Identifying negative self-talk, I think it's better to do this list in handwriting, not on the computer. This makes a stronger connection with your physical self, your neurons, your psyche and intuition, which is important here. What your body does, your subconscious learns from.

Try folding a piece of lined paper in half lengthwise, and then unfold it. Down the left side, write a list of those self-limiting statements you've been thinking and saying to yourself, such as, "I don't have time to take a vacation" or, "I will never get into shape" or, "I won't be able to earn enough money."

Take some time with this. Spend a few days listening to what you're saying to yourself, observing the self-sabotaging "weeds" clogging your subconscious thinking. Ask a friend to listen, too. Add every negative self-talk statement to your list as it comes up.

After you think you've written them all, wait. More will come. As you empty out the top layer in your mind, the next layer will be revealed and released. Since most of us are unaware of this repetitive voice poisoning our thoughts and words, this is a very valuable exercise.

If you're having difficulty accessing this layer of your mind and thoughts, there are coaches and therapies available that can help bring this level of your inner life to light with you. For many people this work can be more powerful than it may seem at first, and there's no harm finding a good coach.

2) Create Affirmations from the Self-Talk and Beliefs—Create New Dreams for Your Life

You are now going to write some new statements. You may feel some (or a lot of) resistance as you do this! Maybe you won't believe a thing you write. Perhaps you'll feel discouraged. You'll probably think it's weird but just humor me on this one—like I did with my coach.

Down the right side of your paper, across from each left-side statement, write a new one that transforms that negative statement into a positive:

"I don't have time to take a vacation" becomes, "I am now easily making time for rest, recreation and vacation!"

"I will never get into shape" becomes, "I am getting into better shape every day!"

"I won't be able to earn enough money" becomes, "An abundance of funds (and every good thing) flows to me easily and effortlessly... and I am grateful!"

These new statements must be in the present tense. Write "I am now..." rather than "I will be..." or "I'm going to be...". Don't use the word "try" because "I'm trying" is a self-perpetuating statement that never quite gets there. Also, don't use "I want..." which implies starting from lack or need. Remember, you're telling your subconscious what to act upon, so be specific and leave no room for confusion.

To get around your disbelief about writing something that feels untrue and seems impossible, you can write things like "I am *learning to*...." and "I am *getting better at*....". It's still in the present tense and still a positive affirmation. Something like, "I am *getting better at* saving money" might feel truer to you than "I am good at saving money."

Now, write down ten big dreams that you have for your life. Imagine you have accomplished them in the present, and imagine how this makes you feel—how proud you are and the sense of accomplishment you have. Write these down beginning with "I am." For example, "I am healthy and in my prime" and "I am a money magnet—money comes to me easily and it multiplies."

3) Begin Using These Affirmations

Fold the paper in half again. Never again read the left side. Ignore it forever!

Post your new affirmations with the positive statements where you'll see it often—on your bedroom mirror or on the fridge, for instance. Read your affirmations two to three times a day. Saying them out loud is an even more powerful way to anchor them into the subconscious. You are transforming your thinking!

If you catch yourself thinking or saying any of your old (negative) beliefs, simply stop yourself. Transform them into the positive, right then and there.

Ask your family and friends to help by simply pointing out any negative self-descriptions when they hear you saying them. When they do, transform the negative to a positive immediately and say the new statement aloud to them. You're literally transforming your mind. Side benefit: you're helping your family and friends transform in the process!

4) Watch the Magic Unfold!

The magic *will truly happen* as you perform these first three tasks. I've done this ever since I learned how and, I promise you, it absolutely works. I am blessed with a good and happy life and things generally go my way. I believe it's because I do this affirmation work regularly.

Soon you will not only *say* you're good at handling money (or whatever your issue is) but you'll also begin to *believe* it and—here's the magic—one day you'll notice that you *are* good at it!

The negative statements will gradually disappear from your mind and the new ones will appear. It's a process. I have found that some things change quickly and some take longer. I also found that some of the things I thought I wanted no longer held my interest, so I took them off my list.

I enjoy the challenges of being a triathlete. A while ago, I added this affirmation to my list: "I am a world-class athlete." Within two months, I received an unexpected letter from the USA Triathlon Association telling me I had qualified to compete in the National Championships.

IT WORKS! ☑

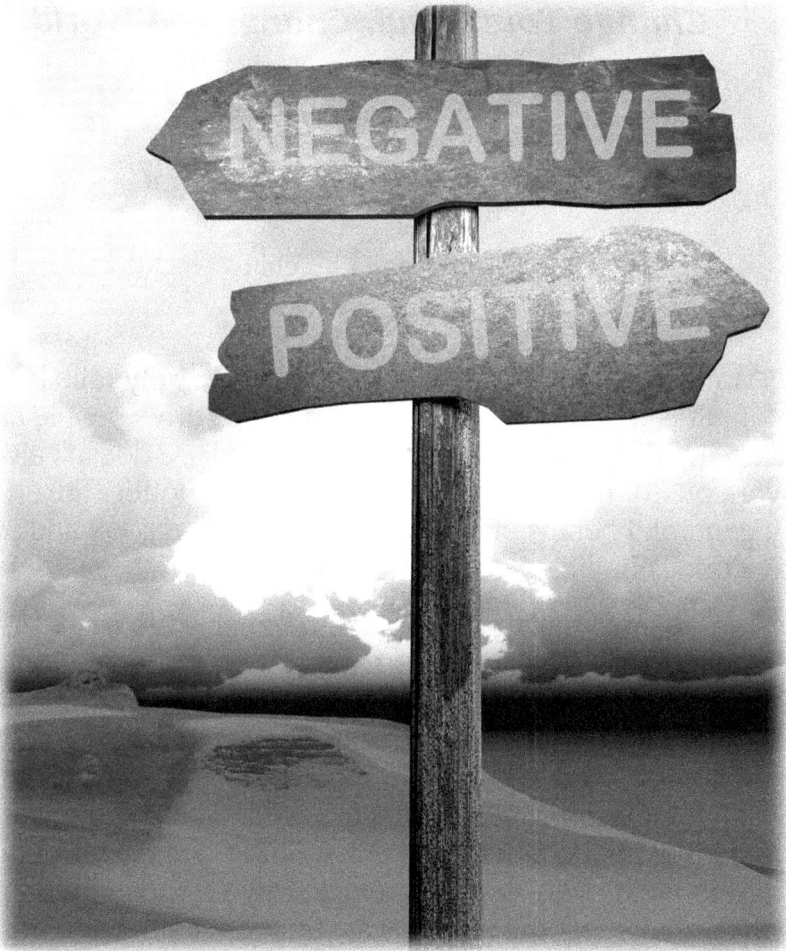

7

Choosing
the Positive

CHAPTER 7

CHOOSING THE POSITIVE—
Change Your Mind, Change the World

*"A pessimist sees the difficulty
in every opportunity;
an optimist sees the opportunity
in every difficulty."*

—Winston Churchill

I am a naturally positive person. Are you? My fallback default is thinking positively. I sometimes drive people crazy with my optimistic attitude. And truthfully, it doesn't always work out for me—like the time I bought that lottery ticket! But in general, I believe it's better to focus on the good and positive things in life.

Positive thinking really does change your brain—not in some magical, "spooky action at a distance" kind of way, but in a real, physical way. The science is called neuroplasticity. It means that your thoughts can change the structure and function of your brain. The idea was first introduced by William James in 1890. He was believed to be one of the most influential philosophers the United States has ever produced, but his ideas were soundly rejected by scientists, who uniformly believed the brain was unchangeable and rigidly mapped out, with certain parts of the brain controlling certain functions. They believed that if a part of the brain is dead or damaged, the function associated with it is altered or lost. Well, it appears they were wrong.

Neuroplasticity now enjoys wide acceptance as scientists are proving the brain is endlessly adaptable and dynamic. It has the power to change its own structure, even for those with severe neurological damage. People with problems like strokes, cerebral palsy, and mental illness can retrain other areas of their brains through repetitive mental and physical activities to take over other functions of their body. So, what does this have to do with positive thinking and with you? It means that repetitive positive thought and positive activity can rewire your brain and strengthen brain areas that stimulate positive feelings.

Professor Barbara Fredrickson is a social psychologist from the University of North Carolina at Chapel Hill, and has been a researcher in human emotions for the past 25 years. She suggests that positivity is the mindset that helps produce emotions such as joy, amusement, happiness, serenity, gratitude and inspiration. She says:

"Negative emotions really hit us like a sledgehammer. They are much more intense and attention-grabbing than our positive emotions, which are comparably subtler... We have an ingrained negativity bias.

I think of positive emotions as nutrients. In the same way that we need to eat a variety of fruits and vegetables to be healthy, we need a variety of positive emotions in our daily experience to help us become more resourceful versions of ourselves."

Imagine two sales people who receive the same rejection from a customer. The first thinks, "I'm such a failure! I always do poorly at this job. I can't do anything right!" The second thinks, "This customer was difficult! Oh well, it's just one customer in one sale. I tend to do well in sales." These two are exhibiting two types of what psychologists call, "explanatory styles." Explanatory styles reflect three attributions that a person forms about a recent event. Did it happen because of me (internal) or something or someone else (external)? Will this always happen to me (stable) or can I change what caused it (unstable)? Is this something that affects all aspects of my life (pervasive) or was it a solitary occurrence (limited)? Pessimistic people tend to view problems as internal, unchangeable, and pervasive; whereas optimistic people are the opposite—viewing circumstances as external, changeable, and limited.

Pessimism has been linked with depression, stress, and anxiety (Kamen & Seligman, 1987), whereas optimism has been shown to serve as a protective factor against depression, as well as several other serious medical conditions, including coronary heart disease (Tindle, et. al., 2009). Optimistic mothers even deliver healthier, heavier babies (Lobel, DeVincent, Kaminer, & Meyer, 2000).

Optimism seems to have a tremendous number of benefits. But just like getting physically fit or improving our nutrition, changing to a positive outlook takes time and effort. Here are seven things I do that help me keep a positive outlook:

1) Start the day with a positive affirmation.

Belief consists in accepting the affirmations
of the soul; unbelief, in denying them.

—Ralph Waldo Emerson

How you start your morning lays the foundation for the rest of your day. Think back on a morning where you started off the day with not enough sleep, had a fight with your spouse, or woke up from a negative dream. It had a negative impact on your day, didn't it? Now think back to a morning when the opposite was the case—your mindset really does make a difference. Remember what we talked about in the last chapter?

Recently a buddy of mine recommended *The Five-Minute Journal* by Alex Ikonn & UJ Ramdas. It's a quick, daily journal where you list three things you are grateful for, three things that would make your day great, and one daily affirmation. Since I started using it, not only has it started my day off on a positive note, but I am also more focused on my primary mission for the day. For example, today one of the things that would make this day great would be that I added more stories to two chapters in this book. *Voila!* This is my second chapter. What a great day!!

Develop those affirmations, begin your day repeating those to yourself at the beginning, the middle, and the end of your day. It will make a big difference!

2) Focus on the good things, however small.

Your mind is astonishingly powerful.
Focus that power on the good things.

—Ralph Marston

Almost invariably, you're going to encounter obstacles throughout the day—there's no such thing as a perfect day. When you encounter such a challenge, focus on the benefits, no matter how slight or unimportant they may seem. For example, if you get stuck in traffic, think about how you now have time to listen to the rest of your favorite podcast. If the store is out of the food you want to prepare, think about the thrill of trying something new.

3) Find humor in bad situations.

He who laughs, lasts!

—Mary Pettibone Poole

Don't be afraid to laugh at yourself and allow yourself to experience humor in even the direst or most trying of situations. Life can dish out some mean stuff sometimes. If you can remind yourself that this situation will probably make for a good story later on and try to crack a joke about it, you will be in a better mindset to handle the stress of the situation. None of us are perfect, so don't take life's ups and downs too seriously.

Let's say you just got laid off. Imagine the most absurd way you could spend your last day, or the most ridiculous job you could pursue next—like kangaroo handler or bubble-gum sculptor.

4) Turn failures into lessons.

> *The greatest mistake we make is living*
> *in constant fear that we will make one.*

—John Maxwell

Since you aren't perfect, you're going to make mistakes and experience failures in multiple contexts, at multiple jobs, and with multiple people. Instead of focusing on how you failed, think about what you're going to do better next time— turn your failure into a lesson. Conceptualize this in concrete rules. For example, you could come up with three new rules for managing projects when one of yours didn't turn out as planned.

5) Transform negative self-talk into positive self-talk.

> *Finally, brothers, whatever is true,*
> *whatever is noble, whatever is right, whatever is pure,*
> *whatever is lovely, whatever is admirable—*
> *if anything is excellent or praiseworthy—*
> *think about such things.*

—Saint Paul, Philippians 4:8

Negative self-talk can creep up easily and is often hard to notice. You might think, I'm so bad at this, or I shouldn't have tried that. But these thoughts turn into internalized feelings and might cement your conception of yourself. When you catch yourself doing this, stop and replace those negative messages with positive ones. For example, *I'm so bad at this,* becomes *When I get more practice I'll be way better at this.* And the thought, *I shouldn't have tried that,* becomes *That didn't work out as planned—maybe next time.*

6) Focus on the present.

"If you want to be happy, do not dwell in the past,
do not worry about the future,
focus on living fully in the present."

—Roy T. Bennett, *The Light in the Heart*

I'm talking about the present here—not today, not this hour, only this exact moment. You might be getting chewed out by a customer, but what, in this exact moment, is happening that's so bad? Forget the comment he made five minutes ago. Forget what he might say five minutes from now. Focus on this individual moment. In most situations, you'll find it's not as bad as you imagined it to be. Most sources of negativity stem from a memory of a recent event or the exaggerated imagination of a potential future event. These will hold less power if you stay in the present moment.

7) Find positive friends, mentors and co-workers.

"Choosing the people who will be your friends
will be the most important choice you make."

—Dennis Skattum, Rancher (my father)

The people we surround ourselves with will alter the direction of our lives—for good or bad. Make sure you evaluate the impact of the people you choose to associate with in your life. Don't be afraid to cut ties with people who drag you down and are not in alignment with the upward direction of your life. And don't be afraid to seek people out who are already where you want to be.

Life is full of unknown twists and turns. Sometimes things turn out surprisingly good and other times, things can go unimaginably horrific. We don't always know which way life will take us. I believe that if we choose to be optimistic about the future, in general, good things tend to come our way. When the hard knocks come, we just figure out how to deal with them. On the other hand, when we tend to be pessimistic, I believe that, in general, bad things will more often come our way and we will still have to figure out how to deal with them. The way we think creates the way we act and the way we act creates our outcomes. So, I chose optimism. I hope you will too.

Will positive thoughts always be more accurate and closer to the truth? In my opinion, YES! My studies with the Napoleon Hill Foundation have shown me that negative and limiting thoughts and beliefs, especially about oneself, will never lead to productive results. Here's their definition of accurate thinking:

> *Accurate Thinking is the mental process that enables us to identify that which is TRUE and RELEVANT. It is more than critical thinking which is just our ability to analyze the agenda and thoughts of others. Accurate Thinking is concerned with creating new agendas, new thoughts and new visions.*

[www.naphill.org/focus-instructors/accurate-thinking]

☑

8

Time To Learn!

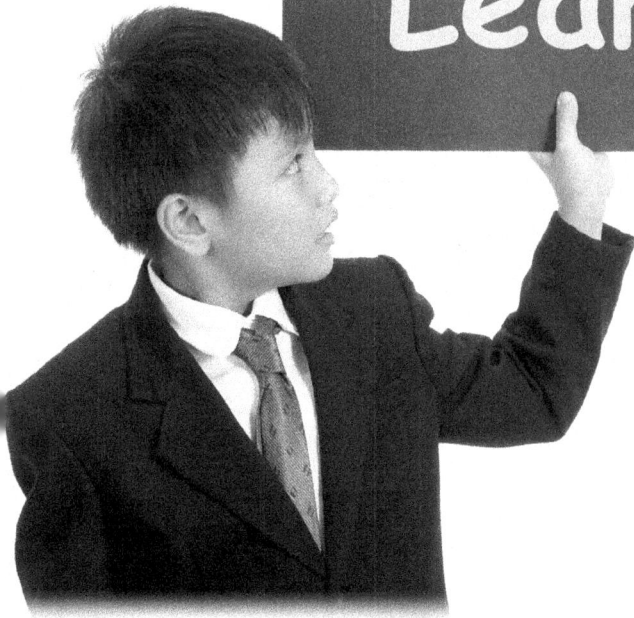

Learning to Grow

CHAPTER 8

LEARNING TO GROW—
Brain Stretcher!

The more that you read,
The more things you will know.
The more that you learn,
The more places you'll go.

—Dr. Seuss, *I Can Read With My Eyes Shut!*

A few years ago, I decided to improve my swimming proficiency. I was comfortable in the water but dog paddling was a gracious description of my swimming style. I wanted to be able to do that thing where you keep your head in the water and spin your arms around like a windmill, with majestic movement and grace. How hard could it be?

So, I bought a six-month pass to the local pool, a pair of goggles, and jumped in! That first day is etched in my soul like a bad dream. I stayed in the shallow end and attempted to swim across the short width of the pool. I shoved off with both my feet and started the windmill thing with my arms.

At first, I thought I was doing okay, but then my head hit the bottom of the pool causing my lungs to inhale— water! I was finally able to get my feet under me and came up gasping, choking and spitting that stinking chlorinated pool water. The sixteen-year-old lifeguard jumped off her guard tower, fearing for my life, grabbed me around the chest, and told me I should get some swimming lessons. I still count this as one of the most embarrassing moments of my life—but I did take her advice and got some swimming lessons. Today I am a fairly good swimmer. I compete in 1,000-meter to 2-mile swimming events. All because I learned something new.

I think that a challenged, stimulated brain is key to having a vibrant life, especially as we age. As many of us are preparing for the retirement years, news keeps coming in that staying active and keeping our brains constantly engaged helps to stave off mental and physical decline and disease. This has many of us asking how best to do so. The simple answer is: *Keep Learning to Grow.*

Nancy Merz Nordstrom, author of *Learning Later, Living Greater*, advocates life-long learning. She shares, "When you look at the benefits gained from keeping your mind sharp, it's incredible. Lifelong learning is like a health club for your brain. And an active mind can stimulate physical activity and keep your spirits high. It's an all-around fantastic tool for better health."

Here are some of the main areas of your life that will improve when you keep learning new things as you grow older:

1) Economic

Most of us will end up switching jobs numerous times; researchers say it will be anywhere from two to seven times! And even those of us fortunate (or unfortunate) enough to stay in the same job for a long time will see the nature of the work we do shift continually. To thrive economically, you simply must keep learning.

I'd argue, too, that it will be increasingly important to be well-rounded, to have a sense of perspective, and to be able to leverage a variety of learning experiences and multiple skill sets into generating new ideas and ways of doing things. The more you know, the more money you will make. I can't say enough about Toastmasters International and highly recommend you find a local club, visit toastmasters.org. You will learn to communicate better and to lead effectively, which inevitably leads to career advancement and a more successful life. (It has worked wonders for me.)

2) Intellectual

I use the term "intellectual" broadly. It doesn't mean that you need to be a bearded professor; rather, that learning to grow increases your knowledge and your ability to use that knowledge in diverse and meaningful ways. Learning to grow opens, stimulates and enhances your mind. I believe it fuels creativity and innovation.

At the same time, learning to grow is an approach to living life consciously and deliberately, rather than being guided purely by instinct, emotion, or the desires of others.

3) Social

Learning sparks social engagement. We often connect with others (like that young lifeguard in the pool) because we want to learn from them and with them. I think that people with strong social connections tend to be happier and live longer. The same goes for societies.

And, as the psychologist John Dewey famously wrote: *Education is not preparation for life; education is life itself.* Lifelong learning is important as an element of democratic societies and your learning efforts support the greater good.

4) Spiritual

Learning new things feeds the spirit. It gives us purpose, a focus, and it fuels our sense of fulfillment. Bob Dylan famously wrote, "Proves to warn that he not busy being born is busy dying," from "It's Alright, Ma (I'm Only Bleeding)." You could easily substitute "learning to grow" for "being born" in this line. Philosophers since well before Dylan have felt the same. Pick up a book on spiritual teachings, whatever your preference, and the inspiration you'll gain and enrich your life and those around you. My spiritual connection is the most prominent "fuel" that propels me forward in a quest for health and a joyful life.

5) Adaptability

Our lives and our society are in a state of constant flux. Often as we age we might feel like the proverbial "old dog that can't learn new tricks." That's not true at all, says Nancy Nordstrom: "Lifelong learning enables us to keep up with society's changes—especially the technological ones. A learning environment with our peers not only makes it possible to stay abreast of change, it also makes it fun." Almost every city offers inexpensive adult-education programs where you can find fun, well-taught courses on all kinds of subjects. Check one out!

Now you might be asking, "What can I do, specifically, to learn to grow?" Glad you asked! Here are a few things I try to do to keep myself in a state of always learning:

• Read Widely and Often

Buy newspapers, search for things online that you want to know more about, ask your friends for books they found helpful or inspirational—above all, stay curious! If you want to find in-depth research on a topic, use Google Scholar to find academic papers. Delve into a topic and don't stop until you have exhausted it! I subscribe to Audible.com, which gives me access to two new books a month. It works great for me to listen to a book as I am driving. I can chose almost any kind of book I want and learn and grow from it. Also, with my subscription to Audible.com comes a free daily subscription to the Wall Street Journal. I usually listen to that daily. It's usually a 30-to-45-minute-long summary of the paper. It works well for me to listen to this during my drive time.

• Keep Smart Company

Reach out to contacts that you admire. You will be surprised that most influential people want to spend time with you, helping you out on your journey. Make sure to keep in touch with people you have met who have inspired you to learn. Cultivate a circle of friends who enjoy stimulating conversations and an array of viewpoints.

I will never forget the day I decided to contact a man who was in my mind, a business master far above my pay grade. I remember being totally intimidated about calling him and asking him for a cup of coffee. It took me 2 days to build up the courage to call him. I thought for sure that he would say he was way too busy to meet with a peasant like me. When I did finally call him, the conversation went something like this: Me—"Hi Tom, my name is Dave Skattum. I have some ideas about a new business I would like to run by you and was wondering if you would have an hour of time to spend with me over a cup of coffee sometime." Tom said, "Sure, when do you want to meet?" I nearly dropped my phone! Today Tom is one of my best friends and has helped me grow exponentially. What's the old saying—"You have not because you ask not?"

• Teach Others

You don't need to join the teaching profession to help people learn. Teaching others what you know will also help ensure that you really understand something well. Volunteer for a local kid's program like Big Brothers Big Sisters of America, or in your church youth group. Kids everywhere need your knowledge and wisdom.

• **Make and Check Off Your Bucket List**

Many times, there are amazing things to explore right in your backyard, or not too far away. Make a list of dreams you have and things you want to accomplish. Once you've developed a list, then you can decide what is the best option to follow and who to enjoy your adventures with!

Try this: A few years ago, I wrote out a bucket list of (in my mind) unimaginable things that I wanted to accomplish. Then I converted them to affirmations. For example, one of the things on the bucket list was to write a book. So, I began to tell myself that, "My writings are impacting the world." Here I am writing my first book and my hope is that it will change the world—amazing!

• **Find a Personal Learning Environment**

Understanding how to learn is an invaluable skill. Opportunities, environments and groups that foster learning are everywhere—local theater, community gardens, volunteering, clubs and organizations, serving on committees and boards—anywhere where you're actively contributing. When you find the learning environment that suits you best, you'll be on your way to discovering new knowledge. You will be surprised how inspired you will get when you're with a group of friends that share your interests.

• **Experiment with New Ways of Learning**

Trying a variety of ways to learn will help you to find the way that works best for you. Drawing diagrams, watching documentaries, creating mind maps and playing music when studying are some alternative ways you can experiment with learning.

• Join a Study Group

Find forums and study groups online where you can collaborate and learn from people with varying experiences. Take insights from a variety of sources and apply them to your own knowledge search. Form a mastermind group in your local area with similar goals to explore new ideas and try out new things.

• Find a Job that Encourages Learning and Collaboration

Most professional roles include some degree of learning, whether it's on-the-job training, seminars or other educational encouragement. Pursuing a career in an evolving area will ensure that you are constantly learning and developing your skill set.

• Make Learning a Priority!

Don't just keep saying "one day." Make today that day! Whether you're a teacher, a student, or a professional, make learning a priority in your life. If you wait for it to find you, you may limit the amount of information you know, plus your ability to attain this knowledge over the long-term.

I believe there is great value in continually learning to grow. You will improve your well-being, contribute more effectively to society, and live a longer, healthier, happier life. ☑

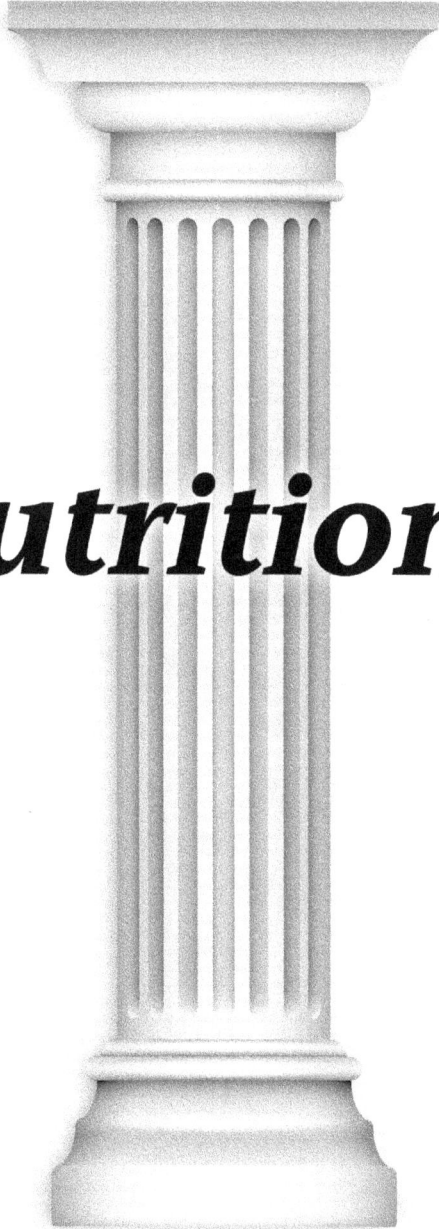

Second Pillar

Nutrition

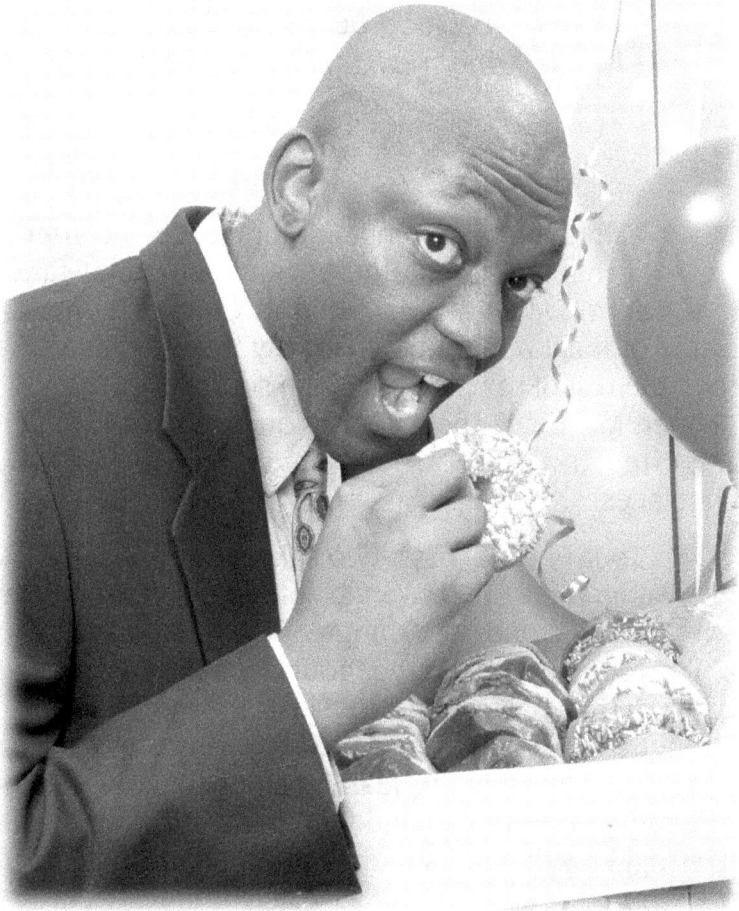

9

The Death
of Dieting

CHAPTER 9

THE DEATH OF DIETING—
The Birth of Good Nutrition

*Let food be thy medicine
and medicine be thy food.*

—Hippocrates

When that lightning bolt hit me, i.e., my friend having his leg amputated because of complications with diabetes as described in Chapter 1, my diet consisted of meat and potatoes for my "healthy meals," and fast food the rest of the time. My main source of hydration was Dr. Pepper. My idea of better nutrition was to NOT super-size it. I sported the type of belly that made it hard to see my shoelaces.

Today I eat at least two salads and 6–7 servings of fruit every day. I've lost 55 pounds. Joint pain and severe episodes with kidney stones are things of the past. I have gained the ability to run around in the mountains like I did when I was in high school. I have energy that lasts the day and good physical strength and vitality. I am not a health expert—just inspired to pass on to you what I've learned along the way. This has been a seven-year journey filled with many ups and downs. I had to struggle with understanding nutrition and how it affects my body; I had no clue. I had to deal with lifestyle and cultural changes—converting to a plant-based diet on a Montana ranch raised some eyebrows—and not the cattle's! And I had to and still am dealing with food addictions—more on that later in Chapter 12.

Let me tell you what I think I did right, and then explain where I failed. First, I decided I had to do something, or I knew that I would be in the hospital soon. Making that choice to change was the first important step I took. The second thing I did right was to start using healthy affirmations. I would say to myself, "I am a lean, mean 155-pound machine because I eat right and exercise daily." I believe this began to set my subconscious onto the right path to discovering good nutrition. By the way, I am still about 25 pounds away from that goal of 155.

The second thing I did right was to educate myself about what good nutrition looks like for me. A major influence was Dr. Joel Fuhrman and his many books and programs.

The third thing I did right was to start hanging out with people who would be an encouragement to me in my search for good physical health (new friends, coaches, fellow strugglers, doctors and natural-health practitioners) and improved mental, emotional and spiritual health as well.

The first thing I did wrong was to think of my new eating habits as a diet, because when I would get close to where I wanted to be with my health, I would quit that pesky diet. The weight came back on; the joint pain came back; I lost energy and vitality. I began to understand that I had to make this new way of eating a way of life.

The second thing I did wrong was to have an unrealistic expectation of how long it would take to drop my excess weight. I did too much too fast. This kind of thinking leads to dangerous, yo-yo weight loss. It took me 30 years to put on the extra 70 pounds; it needed to be ok to be patient and take a few years to get rid of it. Better to take it slow and steady.

The third thing I did wrong was to focus on weight loss. Now, the primary thing for me is simply being a healthy, well-balanced person. It took a lot of pressure off and it's now a life-long journey, not just a weight-loss-through-dieting goal. I get to enjoy the journey now—all the positive things I do naturally and easily contribute to losing and maintaining a healthy weight.

THE BAD NEWS FIRST

The main thing that's important for you to know about poor nutrition (and you probably already DO know this) is that it can impair your daily health and well-being, and reduce your ability to lead an enjoyable and active life. In the short term, poor nutrition can contribute to stress, tiredness, and a diminished capacity to work. Over time, it can contribute to developing major health risks, such as:

- Being overweight or obese
- Tooth decay
- High blood pressure
- High cholesterol
- Heart disease and stroke
- Type-2 diabetes
- Osteoporosis
- Some cancers
- Eating disorders
- Depression

What you need to know about being overweight is that carrying excess weight increases the risk of many health problems (www.niddk.nih.gov), including:

- Type-2 diabetes
- High blood pressure
- Heart disease and strokes
- Certain types of cancer
- Sleep apnea
- Osteoarthritis
- Fatty-liver disease
- Kidney disease

So SAD: The Standard American Diet

Here's what I have learned about the standard American diet. The typical diet of most Americans is far too high in meat, dairy, the wrong fats, sugar, as well as too much refined processed foods, and junk foods. The shift in Western diets to include more animal-sourced foods, and more sugar and corn syrup happened especially quickly after World War II, with the development of industrial farming and food processing practices.

The Standard American Diet includes a low intake of fruits and vegetables. A 2010 report from the U.S. Centers for Disease Control showed that, overall, only one US state improved on vegetable-and-fruit consumption compared to such consumption ten years earlier. A study showing compliance with 2005 U.S. Department of Agriculture dietary guidelines showed only one-fourth of Americans ate at least one fruit serving a day, while only about 1 in 10 ate the recommended minimum amount of vegetables. The average amount of kale each American eats per week is about half a teaspoon. Americans eat so few foods rich in antioxidants that beer represents the fifth-largest source of antioxidants in the standard American diet! The total percentage of calories from foods that are rich in phytonutrients (plant nutrients) in the standard American diet rates at about 11 percent.

Switching to a plant-based, nutrition-oriented diet can help prevent and even reverse some of the top killer diseases in the Western world and can be more effective than medication and surgery. Even after years of eating the standard American diet, it's possible to reduce the risk of chronic, degenerative diseases simply by eating healthier.

In an article at TheSisterRap.com, research studies have found potential links between the standard American diet and risks of the following diseases and conditions in men:

- Acidosis, which contributes to progressive muscle loss
- Acne
- Greater risk of Alzheimer's disease
- Greater risk of atherosclerosis
- Greater risk for breast pain
- Higher levels of IGF-1, a growth hormone associated with cancer risk
- Thicker carotid arteries, linked to cardiovascular mortality risk
- Elevated levels of bad cholesterol
- Increased absorption of endotoxins
- Greater risk of enlarged prostate and heart attack
- Dangerous types of free radicals
- Greater risk of heart disease
- Unhealthy inflammation and oxidation
- Greater risk of inflammatory bowel disease
- Reduction of inner-blood-vessel lining functioning
- Declining kidney function
- Lower-back pain and problems
- Worsening of lung function and asthma control
- Greater risk of pancreatic cancer
- Greater risk of prostate cancer
- Obesity
- Small stools and colon build-up

What I have learned about dieting is that it's a lot like starving, physically. It's like putting your body into that same state that it would be in if you were literally starving to death. I think there are four major reasons why dieting doesn't work:

1) **Neurological.** When you are dieting, you become more likely to notice food. Basically, your brain becomes overly responsive to food—especially to tasty-looking food. But you don't just notice it— it begins to look more appetizing and tempting. It has increased reward value. The thing you're trying to resist becomes harder to resist. So already, if you think about it, it's not fair!

2) **Hormonal Changes.** It's the same kind of thing. As you lose body fat, the number of different hormones in your body changes. The level of hormones that help you feel full decreases, while the level of hormones that make you feel hungry increases. So, you become more likely to feel hungry, and less likely to feel full, given the same amount of food. Again, completely unfair.

3) **Biological Changes.** As Traci Mann from the University of Minnesota's Health and Eating Lab explains, "When dieting, your metabolism slows down. Your body uses calories in the most efficient way possible. Which sounds like a good thing, and it would be good thing if you're starving to death. But it isn't a good thing if you're trying to lose weight, because when your body finds a way to run itself on fewer calories there tends to be more calories left over, and those get stored as fat, which is exactly what you don't want to happen!"

When I am on an extended fast, the first few days the weight drops off fast but then my body begins to realize that food might not be coming that day and changes things up about how it uses energy. It becomes much more efficient with what it has. Same with starvation dieting. It might work good for a while but after a period of time it gets hard and it seems like a bottle of water will add a pound of fat.

4) **Food Addiction.** This often involves the uncontrollable pursuit of a mood change by eating unhealthy food. The addictive foods excessively stimulate the reward centers of the brain, creating an almost irresistible craving for them. People who suffer from food addictions find that they get a high when they eat their trigger foods, followed by a low when they are not properly digesting them, creating a vicious cycle and a desire for more trigger foods. The condition is chronic, progressive and—given the unhealthy nature of the addictive foods—it's dangerous and potentially fatal!

NOW, FOR THE GOOD NEWS!

Wait! There's hope and a path to good health! Here are four steps I took and I believe they will work well for you, too. First, you make the decision to change your nutrition—hopefully NOT waiting until the doctor is there with the amputation saw! Second, you change your beliefs about yourself and nutrition, and start to retrain your subconscious through affirmations. Third, you educate yourself about nutrition. Hey, you're reading this, so that's a great start! Fourth, you build a support team—and yes, I'm already on it!

1) Make a Decision to Change Your Nutrition

You already know that what you're doing for nutrition is not working. The food you're eating is making you fat and unhealthy—and that's only the part of the iceberg that you can see! You must start with, "I have got to make a change!" Don't worry at this point where your decision will take you; just decide that you are going to make a change for the better.

Your path will be different than mine. It will wind along different roads and through many ups and downs, but the important thing is that you decide—in your mind, heart and soul—to change!

For me, this happened when my friend had his leg amputated because of diabetes, and I knew I was heading in that direction. I also have a strong desire to live a long active, healthy life. I watched my grandmother die a slow, demented death that landed her in a mental hospital near the end of her life. A gruesome experience. I don't want those experiences for myself or those who would have to go through it with me. I had to weigh out the options; was I going to continue with the fast food route and norms of society or was I going to change my nutrition and buck the system? I decided on the latter. You need to decide what's important to you. Be a leader and make the decision to change your nutrition.

2) Change Your Beliefs About Yourself and Nutrition

Now is the time to activate those affirmations. Replace negative thoughts like, "I will never be healthy," or "I could never eat that way," with, "I will get to my ideal weight because I am eating right!" and "I will do those activities that I love!" You must put your subconscious in a position where it will naturally begin to find health and nutrition solutions for you. You do this by making positive statements to yourself. Another approach is to pray to God for direction and answers. I always do both—and they work.

3) Educate Yourself About Nutrition

Now start to do research into what it means for you to eat healthy. For the reasons mentioned above, I encourage you to stay away from dieting plans. Find a healthy way to eat. You can start slowly at first, but make it a lifestyle change that eventually becomes permanent.

You become what you eat—the nutrition you put in your mouth creates the cells that build your body and that will impact your health and vitality in the future. Our bodies need both macro- and micronutrients. Macronutrients are the structural and energy-giving caloric components of our foods that most of us are familiar with. They include carbohydrates, fats and proteins. Micronutrients are the *vitamins, minerals, trace elements, phytochemicals, and antioxidants* that are essential for healthy cells. The SAD diet has too much of macronutrients and too little of micronutrients.

This is at the core of what is causing us to be overweight and unhealthy. The quantity of macronutrients in our food (and their *quality*, i.e., healthy calories versus empty calories) give us way too many carbohydrates, sugars and fat, and the lack of micronutrients (eating too many dead foods that are bankrupt in nutrient value) is also causing us to be unhealthy. *(See the chart below.)*

Caloric Density

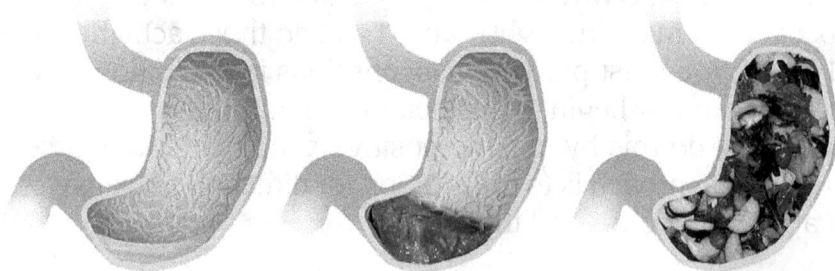

| 400 Calories of Oil | 400 Calories of Beef | 400 Calories of Vegetables |

Stretch receptors are located throughout the stomach. When they are triggered by food, they send signals to your brain to tell you to stop eating. With high fiber, whole plant foods, you can eat the most quantity for the least amount of calories.

© 2012 Julieanna Hever, MS, RD, CPT • www.PlantBasedDietitian.com   Illustration by Sherri Nestorowich • www.sherrinest.wix.com/art

Above all, choose nutrition that has a high nutrient to calorie ratio. *Men's Journal*, in an article entitled, "The Best and Worst Foods on the ANDI Scale," said it this way:

"One of the best ways to prevent weight gain and disease is to maximize your micronutrients. Dr. Fuhrman recommends what he calls the Nutritarian Diet—eating foods with the most micronutrients per calorie. Since most micronutrients aren't listed on labels, he created the 1,000-point Aggregate Nutrient Density Index (ANDI), which ranks foods based on micronutrient concentration. Rankings are based on a 1,000-point scale, with 1,000 indicating that a food contains the highest number of micronutrients per calorie."

[MensJournal.com/expert-advice/the-best-and-worst-foods-on-the-andi-scale-20130403]

You can find this information online or order Dr. Fuhrman's book, *Nutritarian Handbook & ANDI Food Scoring Guide.* Coming up, Chapter 11 on the ANDI Food Scores.

Here is how I choose my nutrition today:

- I avoid processed and refined foods (sugar, oils, spreads, refined grains, etc.)

- I eat only whole foods. (Hint: it looks like a food, rather than a can or a box.)

- I avoid excessive animal-product intake, limiting it to only a few ounces a day. I have switched from the fattier choices: like from beef to fish or chicken, and from eggs to foods like greens, beans, onions and garlic, mushrooms, berries, seeds and nuts.

- I limit table-salt intake. However, note that high-quality mineral salts can be found at the health-food store that will greatly increase your micronutrient intake.

- I fill a significant portion of my meal with raw and/

or lightly cooked, whole-plant foods (vegetables, legumes, nuts, seeds, and fruits). However, note that there are schools of food combining that advise that fruits are better eaten alone, because they digest much quicker.

• I find a good, live, green superfood supplement product that you enjoy and add it to fortify a daily smoothie or green drink. (More about superfoods in the fasting chapter.)

4) Build a Support Team

Making these changes is a radical, life-altering process. I couldn't have made it through the changes I did without the support of a bunch of people that encouraged and helped me along. It's so important, when you are making big changes in your life, that you have people around you who will walk through it with you. This is not the time to be the Lone Ranger! Build a team, get a coach, recruit a buddy, sit down with your family and get them onboard with you—they'll love being included. There are specialized forums and groups to join, including ours at: The4PillarsOfMensHealth.com.

Good nutrition is so critical to your health and vitality, but dieting doesn't work and we already have such a large amount of opposition to eating right in our past and in our culture. So, let the whole idea of dieting die. And now, let's wake up, man up, make some good decisions, stand out from the crowd, and get healthy. ☑

10

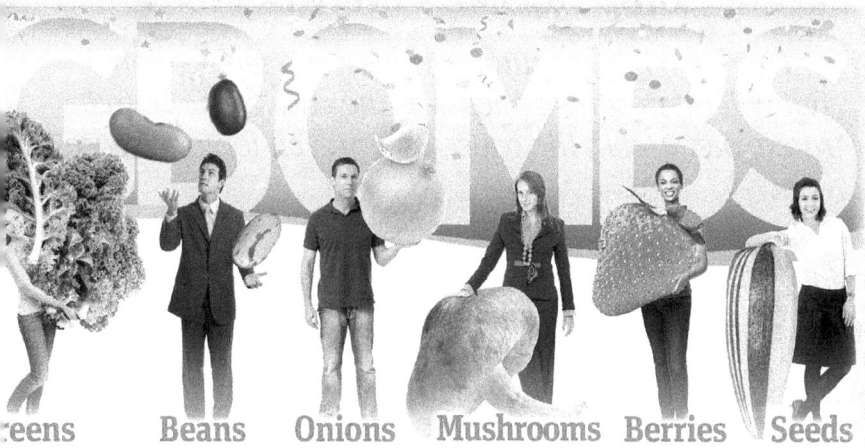

reens   Beans   Onions   Mushrooms   Berries   Seeds

TAKE THE CHALLENGE!

*Eat
These
Foods*

CHAPTER 10

EAT THESE FOODS—
Drop GBOMBS Every Day!

*The doctor of the future will give no medication,
but will interest his patients in the care of the human
frame, diet and in the cause and prevention of disease.*

—Thomas Edison

So many "diet" programs tell you what NOT to eat. I believe there are so many good foods that we should be adding to our daily meals—so why focus on the negative? When we make excellent nutritional choices, most of our health and weight issues disappear. Every day, we should eat foods that nourish and heal our bodies. Much of what I learned about GBOMBS comes from the great mind of Dr. Fuhrman. I recommend any of his books and his website: DrFuhrman.com.

Todd's story from Dr. Fuhrman's website states that his arthritis pain is much better without having to take the toxic drug his doctor had prescribed, and he lost 58 pounds.

"When I started the Nutritarian program my blood pressure was averaging about 138/90, and I was taking blood pressure medication. Two weeks into the program, I was averaging 105/68. I dropped my medication, thinking it might rise dramatically, but it did not. I am a very healthy level of 117/72 on an everyday basis now without meds.

It has also helped me with my autoimmune disease, psoriatic arthritis. My joint pain and inflammation have subsided. Just a month before starting the program, my dermatologist was desperately trying to get me to take Humira, a potentially very dangerous drug. My arthritis pain is also disappearing and I started Bikram Yoga classes five days a week. For me, my 58-pound weight loss was a secondary benefit. I wanted to feel better, and I wanted my numbers to be a lot better. I enjoy the weight loss and the positive self-image it has given me, but nothing beats the new energy and the new life that the Nutritarian Diet has given me. Life is definitely good!"

Let me introduce you to GBOMBS—it's an acronym that you can use to remember the best anti-disease and health-promoting foods on the planet. Yes, you should consume these foods every day, and they should make up a large portion of your diet. They are extremely effective at preventing chronic diseases, including cancer, heart disease and diabetes, and they will enhance your health and longevity. Just look at the benefits of eating these highly nutritious foods listed below. Here are some of the incredible benefits you'll receive from dropping each of these GBOMBS every day:

G = Greens
B = Beans
O = Onions & Garlic
M = Mushrooms
B = Berries
S = Seeds

GREENS

Lower Cholesterol—Mustard greens and kale help lower cholesterol.

Preserve Vision Health—Leafy greens—in particular kale, dandelion, mustard greens and Swiss chard—are good sources of carotenoids, lutein, and zeaxanthin, which help filter high-energy light that may cause eye damage.

Help Fuel your Body—A one-cup serving of raw escarole (a broad-leafed endive used in salads) provides

1/10th of your daily needs for vitamin B5 (pantothenic acid). The B vitamins help convert the carbs in food to glucose, which the body can use as a fuel to produce energy.

Boost Bone Health—The slightly bitter taste of many leafy greens is a good sign—it reflects their high levels of calcium, which builds strong bones.

Prevent Colon Cancer—Kale and mustard greens are part of the nutrient-rich Brassica family, which also includes broccoli and cabbage. A study in the *Journal of the American Dietetic Association* in 2011 linked a higher intake of these vegetables with a decreased risk of cancer in the ascending colon.

I get my greens by adding a green mixture to my smoothie in the morning and having a huge green salad for lunch. I usually get my salad from an organic local salad bar and put every kind of green on my salad that they have available.

BEANS

Prevent Heart Disease—Studies have shown that people who eat more legumes have a lower risk of heart disease, and you can partially thank the phytochemicals found in beans, since they protect against it.

Fight Cancer—Beans contain a wide range of cancer-fighting plant chemicals, specifically, isoflavones and phytosterols, which are associated with reduced cancer risk.

Lower Cholesterol—Beans provide the body with soluble fiber, which plays an important role in controlling blood cholesterol levels.

Lose Weight—A serving of beans will help you feel full more quickly, because the rich fiber content fills your stomach and causes a slower rise in blood sugar.

Manage Diabetes—Beans are a diabetes sufferer's superfood! The balance of complex carbohydrates and protein provides a slow, steady source of glucose, instead of the sudden surge that can occur after eating simple carbohydrates (sugars).

I get my beans in a couple ways. At the salad bar, they usually have a selection of garbanzo, kidney and black beans. I alternate them daily. I also get beans in the form of a delicious soup. I am experimenting with a bean burger, but haven't got that nailed down yet.

ONIONS & GARLIC

Prevent Cancer—A study from the National Cancer Institute found that eating ten grams (approximately two teaspoons) or more of garlic, onions, or scallions per day was associated with a statistically significantly lower risk of prostate cancer for the participants in the study.

Detoxify Your Body—Many cancers are thought to be caused by damage to DNA, often induced by environmental toxins. A study conducted at the Fred Hutchinson Cancer Research Center in Seattle found that eating a teaspoon of fresh garlic and a half cup of onions per day increases the levels of a key enzyme that removes toxins in the blood cells.

Lower Cholesterol—While a highly publicized clinical trial at Stanford University found that garlic did not lower cholesterol levels in healthy people with moderately elevated cholesterol, previous studies have indicated that garlic is more likely to produce beneficial effects on cholesterol in women than in men, and in patients with diabetes or heart disease than in healthy individuals.

I get onions from the salad bar, they add lots of flavor to my salad. I always put them on sandwiches that I eat. Garlic is a little trickier for me. Like my editor once told me, garlic is not a good way to make friends and influence people. Currently, I take a garlic supplement. I try to add garlic to foods and do enjoy the flavor it adds. The problem is the effect it has on those around me. There's definitely room for some personal growth for me in this area.

MUSHROOMS

Increase your Vitamin D—Mushrooms are the only fruit or vegetable source of this critical vitamin. Like us humans, mushrooms produce vitamin D when exposed to sunlight.

Boost your Immune System—A study done on mice and published by the American Society for Nutrition found that white-button mushrooms may promote immune function by increasing the production of antiviral and other proteins that are released by cells as they protect and repair the body's tissues.

Get your Antioxidants—When it comes to antioxidants—the substances that fight free radicals, which are the result of oxidation in our body—we're more likely to think of colorful vegetables than neutral-hued mushrooms. But oxygen radical absorbance capacity (ORAC)—a measure of a food's total antioxidants—of cremini (similar to, but slightly larger than, white-button) and Portobello (large) mushrooms were about the same as found in red peppers.

Kick Up your Metabolism—Mushrooms contain loads of vitamin B2 (riboflavin) and vitamin B3 (niacin). B vitamins are vital for turning food (carbohydrates) into fuel (glucose), which the body burns to produce energy. They also help the body metabolize fats and protein. Overall, B-complex vitamins keep our bodies running like well-oiled machines and reduce the effects of stress.

Be Good to your Bladder—Several types of mushrooms are rich in selenium, an essential trace mineral. 100 grams of raw cremini have 47% of your daily need, cooked shiitakes have 45% and raw white-button have 17%. The higher the level of selenium, the lower your risk of bladder cancer. Selenium is also important for cognitive function, a healthy immune system, and fertility for both men and women.

I get my mushrooms from the salad bar. I also like them in soups and burgers. You don't have to eat a large quantity to get the outstanding benefit. It's also better to lightly cook mushrooms as some claim that raw mushrooms have some carcinogenic issues.

BERRIES

Combat Aging—Antioxidants are your best friend to keep Father Time at bay. They help reverse damage done by toxins and free radicals, and help your body defend itself against dangerous pathogens. The berries highest in antioxidants are blueberries, strawberries, cranberries and açai berries.

Boost the Brain—Because they contain such a high amount of phenols, particularly gallic acid, blueberries are known as "neuro-protective agents." And if you consume more blueberries, they slow cognitive decline and improve memory and motor function. The antioxidants in blueberries protect the body from oxidative stress and reduce inflammation.

Fight Cancer—Clinical studies have even discovered that, unlike radiation and chemotherapy strategies, gallic-acid-rich foods like blueberries can kill cancer without harming healthy cells! Blueberries benefit cancer prevention primarily due to their wide range and quantity of antioxidants.

Support Digestion—Being a natural source of soluble and insoluble fiber, blueberries can help regulate your gastrointestinal track by just eating a couple handfuls a day.

Promote Heart Health—Eating strawberries and blueberries together has a superpower tag-team effect that decreases your risk of heart attack by up to 33 percent. Not in season? Buy the frozen ones and add to your smoothies!

Benefit Your Skin—Skin-care products made with blueberry extract are becoming very popular around the world. It's been reported that the wide spectrum of vitamins and minerals help restore hormonal balance, which counteracts acne, making blueberries an excellent home remedy for this.

Aid Weight Loss—Being low in calories, low on the glycemic index, and high in fiber, everyone has these three reasons to eat a variety of berries to lose weight!

Berries are easy for me. I love them and could eat them all day. I put them in my smoothie. I munch on them during the day and add them to my salad. Delicious food and excellent for you.

SEEDS & NUTS

Improve Immunity—Seeds and nuts are packed full of zinc and selenium, which play a crucial role in keeping your immune system healthy and strong. Many people are deficient in these minerals. The top-six healthiest seeds and nuts are: almonds, flaxseeds, pumpkin seeds, walnuts, sesame seeds, and chia seeds.

Promote Good Digestion—Almost all seeds and nuts provide a significant level of dietary fiber, which can have a myriad of effects on our health. Dietary fiber is primarily associated with digestion, as it helps to stimulate the movement of food through your gut.

Protect Your Heart—Most seeds and nuts contain important fatty acids, namely omega-3s, which are the "good" form of cholesterol. By improving the cholesterol balance in your body, you can significantly reduce inflammation in your body and blood vessels.

Strengthen Your Bones & Teeth—All seeds and nuts contain certain levels of key minerals that our bodies need, including phosphorous, calcium, copper, selenium, and zinc. These minerals help prevent age-related diseases like osteoporosis and osteoarthritis. Seeds and nuts can also improve the health of your teeth.

Prevent Chronic Diseases—Seeds and nuts contain an impressive number of phytochemicals, phenolic acids, lignans, omega-3s, vitamins, and other organic acids that act as antioxidants within the body. By eliminating free radicals, these nutrients, found in such diverse quantities in seeds and nuts, can prevent oxidative stress and the onset of chronic disease.

Stimulate Growth & Development—Seeds and nuts contain a wealth of amino acids and plant proteins, both of which are essential for your body's growth and development.

Lower Diabetes Risk—Seeds and nuts are packed with fiber. One of the unsung benefits of dietary fiber is the impact that it can have on diabetes. By regulating the levels of insulin and glucose in the body and by regulating digestive speed, seeds and nuts can prevent the spikes and drops in blood sugar that are so characteristic of diabetes.

Improve Cognitive Ability—Omega-3 fatty acids have even been linked to the stimulation of brain function and cognition, making seeds and nuts impressive brain boosters as well.

Reduce Inflammation—Seeds and nuts can reduce inflammation throughout the body because of their omega-3s, but this is also done through vitamins and minerals, which are in high supply in seeds and nuts.

Lower Anxiety—Some seeds and nuts can affect the neurotransmitters in the brain and balance the hormones in the body, allowing the body to better cope with stress.

I add seeds to my salad and usually have a package of them in my car for when I get an urge to eat something. They are filling and good to eat.

Instead of worrying so much about foods that you shouldn't eat, begin to add more GBOMBS to your meals. You can rest assured that you are building a strong body. Soon you will notice more energy and better health and then you will no longer crave the unhealthy foods you used to eat. There are many varieties of food in each of the GBOMBS categories. Do some research and some taste-testing, and find out for yourself which ones work best for you.

Every day I have what I call a GBOMBS salad. It has every type of food that we discussed in this chapter. I have learned to love these salads and miss them when I don't have one. At 50+ years old I enjoy trail running. Sometimes I am out for 10-12 hours running in the mountains. I credit GBOMBS for building up my health so that I can do these kinds of things.

Give GBOMBS a try. Start by adding the foods you know you will like, and then begin to add all the others. In a few years, you will have a complete body makeover because, after all, "You are what you eat!"

DROP GBOMBS EVERY DAY!! ☑

11

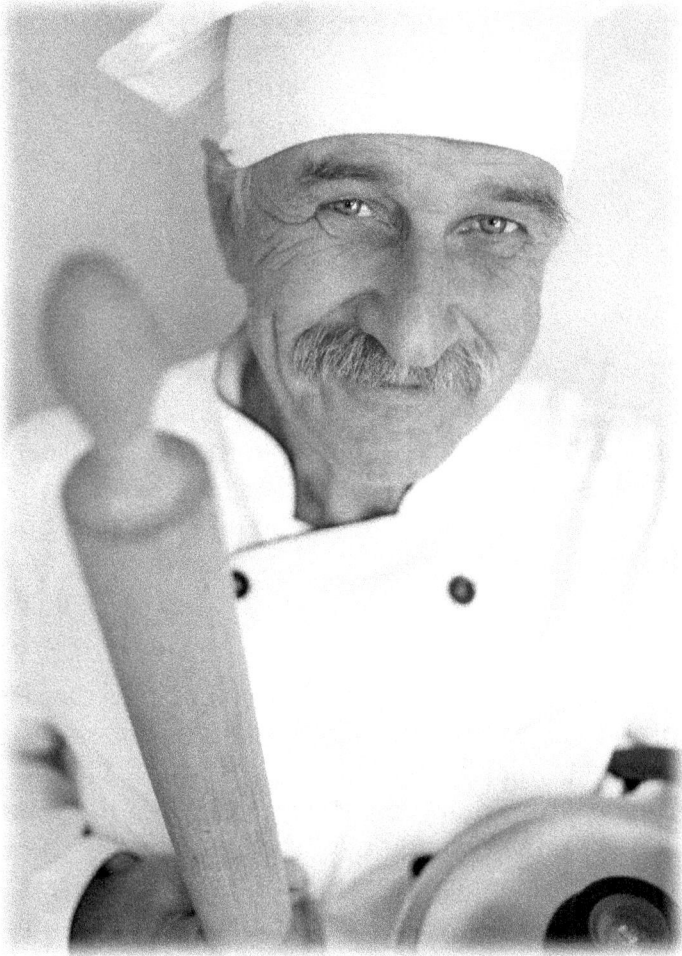

ANDI Food Scores

CHAPTER 11

ANDI FOOD SCORES—
Discovering Excellent Nutrition

*The food you eat can be either the safest
and most powerful form of medicine
or the slowest form of poison.*

—Ann Wigmore, one of America's first holistic-health
practitioners and raw-food advocates

How do you determine what food is best to eat and where do you get it? I remember a day when I became disillusioned about what foods I could eat. I pulled into the gas station where I used to get a corn dog, a bag of chips, and a cola. I knew I couldn't step foot into that building. Then I drove by Wendy's—couldn't stop there. I was so hungry, I went to a food deli and succumbed— fried chicken, jo-jos and onion rings! I ate it all!

I encountered several problems that day. First, I had not preplanned my nutrition for the day. Second, I encountered that tall, thick and very SAD wall—the Standard American Diet. Third, I didn't dig deep enough to find nutritious food. Today I know what I am going to eat during the day. I usually have a fruit and veggie smoothie for breakfast, a salad from a salad bar that I frequent for lunch, and a homemade meal when I get home for dinner. I usually throw in a health bar or nuts during the day if I have a craving.

Our culture is so steeped in poor nutrition today that you can't leave this up to chance, because chances are, you'll only find poor nutrition! In this chapter I will help you identify excellent nutritious food, based on what Dr. Fuhrman, with Eat Right America, has developed, on a scale of 0 to 1000 points. 1000 being the most nutritious and 0 being the least.

For a more in-depth look at this, read *The Nutritarian Handbook* by Dr. Fuhrman.

Good nutrition is high in micronutrients (vitamins, minerals and phytochemicals) and has adequate macronutrition as well (proteins, carbohydrates and fats). The prevailing SAD diet largely contributes to our overweight population and poor health. Lifestyle-related diseases are the most common causes of death, but according to a 2011 poll by Consumer Reports Health, 90% of Americans believe that they eat a healthy diet. At first, I didn't understand myself that whole plant foods were the best for my health. I was led to believe that processed foods labeled "low-fat" or "low-carb," artificially sweetened beverages, pasta, grilled chicken, and olive oil made up a healthy diet.

According to studies done by Dr. Fuhrman, the SAD diet is made up mostly of disease-causing foods, with 30% of our calories coming from animal products and over 55% from processed foods. In addition, 43% of Americans polled reported that they drank at least one sugar-sweetened drink each day, 40% said that they eat "pretty much everything" they want, and 33% of overweight and obese individuals reported that they were at a healthy weight. This highlights the nutritional misinformation that abounds in our society. Most of us have not yet grasped the concept of nutrient density and its importance for health and longevity.

The nutrient density in your body's tissues is proportional to the nutrient density of your diet. Micronutrients fuel proper functioning of the immune system and enable the detoxification and cellular repair mechanisms that protect us from chronic diseases. Dr. Fuhrman coined the term *Nutritarian* to define a diet style that provides a high ratio of micronutrients per calorie and a high level of micronutrient variety. Dr. Fuhrman devised the following simple formula: $H = N/C$ (Health = Nutrients/Calories). This simple equation defines how your health is related to the nutrient density of your diet.

Adequate consumption of micronutrients without excessive caloric intake is the key to achieving excellent health. To illustrate which foods have the highest nutrient-per-calorie density, Dr. Fuhrman created the aggregate nutrient density index, or ANDI. It lets you quickly see which foods are the most health promoting and nutrient-dense.

The ANDI ranks the nutrient value of many common foods based on how many nutrients they deliver to your body for each calorie consumed. Unlike food labels that list only a few nutrients, ANDI scores are based on thirty-four important nutritional parameters. Foods are ranked on a scale of 1 to 1000, with the most nutrient-dense, cruciferous leafy green vegetables scoring 1000.

It is also important to achieve micronutrient diversity, not just a high level of a few isolated micronutrients. Eating a variety of plant foods is essential to good health. It is important to include a wide assortment of plant foods in your diet to obtain the full range of nutritional requirements. Include onions, seeds, mushrooms, berries, beans and tomatoes as well as greens in your diet. They all contribute to the numerator (top number in the ratio) in the $H = N/C$ equation.

Nutrient Scoring Method

Here's a more technical look at how to figure out an ANDI score for your nutrition, and how Dr. Fuhrman comes up with an ANDI score for each food. To determine the ANDI scores, an equal-calorie serving of each food was evaluated. The following nutrients were included in the evaluation: fiber, calcium, iron, magnesium, phosphorus, potassium, zinc, copper, manganese, selenium, vitamin A, beta carotene, alpha carotene, lycopene, lutein, zeaxanthin, vitamin E, vitamin C, thiamin, riboflavin, niacin, pantothenic acid, vitamin B6, folate, vitamin B12, choline, vitamin K, phytosterols, glucosinolates, angiogenesis inhibitors, organosulfides, aromatase inhibitors, resistant starch, resveratrol plus the ORAC score.

ORAC (Oxygen Radical Absorbance Capacity) is a measure of the antioxidant or free-radical-scavenging capacity of a food. For consistency, nutrient quantities were converted from their typical measurement conventions (mg, mcg, IU) to a percentage of their Dietary Reference Intake (DRI). For nutrients that have no DRI, goals were established based on available research and current understanding of the benefits of these factors. To make it easier to compare foods, the raw point totals were converted (multiplied by the same number) so that the highest-ranking foods (leafy green vegetables) received a score of 1000, and the other foods received lower scores accordingly.

Here are the 25 highest ANDI food scores:

Kale	1000
Collards	1000
Mustard greens	1000
Watercress	1000
Swiss chard	895
Bok choy	865
Spinach	707
Arugula	604
Romaine	510
Brussels sprouts	490
Carrots	458
Broccoli rabe	455
Cabbage	434
Broccoli	340
Cauliflower	315
Bell pepper	265
Asparagus	205
Mushrooms	238

For your good health, take a few minutes to evaluate the quality of your current diet and learn which foods you need to consume to improve it. A more comprehensive list of ANDI scores can be found in Dr. Fuhrman's *Nutritarian Handbook & ANDI Food Scoring Guide*. More information can also be found at DrFuhrman.com. ☑

12

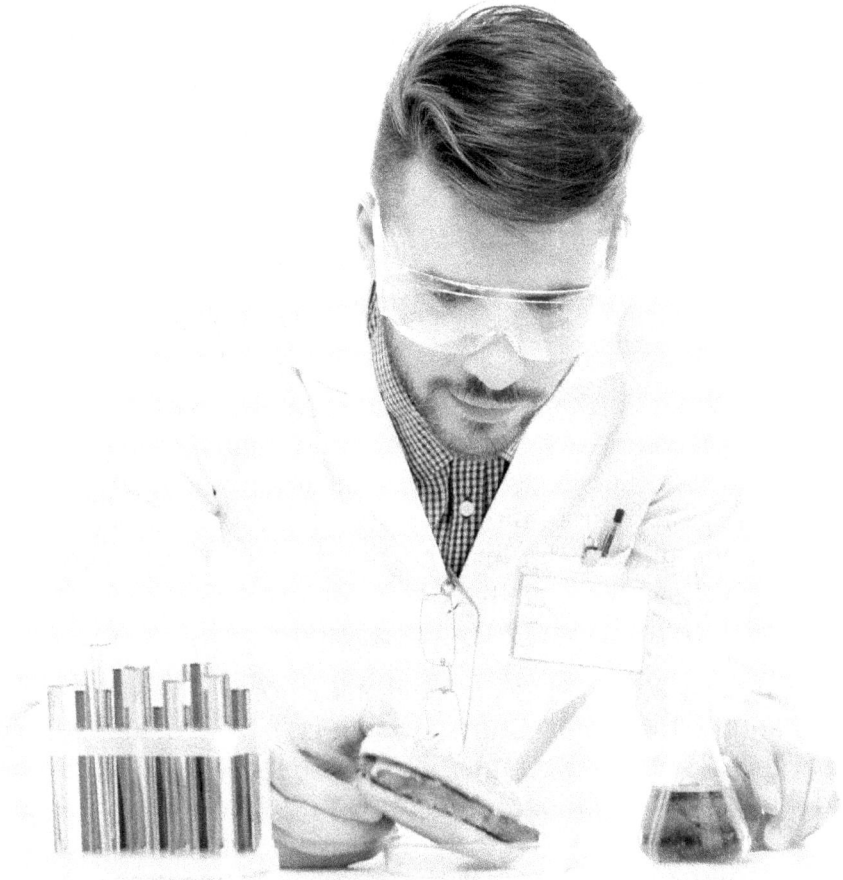

**Toxic Hunger
& Emotional Eating**

CHAPTER 12

TOXIC HUNGER
& EMOTIONAL EATING—
Hand, Mouth & Heart Disease!

*We have these weapons of mass destruction
on every street corner and they're called donuts,
cheeseburgers, french fries, potato chips and junk food.*

—Dr. Joel Fuhrman

Why is it that we have such an urge to eat unhealthy food? We all know that junk food is unhealthy and will cause us problems in the future, but we still can't resist the temptation to grab a chocolate bar, or a corn dog at the gas station, or a sugary doughnut at the grocery store. I believe there are two things going on here: one is toxic hunger and the other is emotional eating.

Toxic hunger is physical addiction to an unhealthy, low-nutrient diet. Emotional eating is eating to suppress or soothe negative emotions, such as stress, anger, fear, boredom, sadness and loneliness. Much of what I believe about these issues is the result of going through enormous struggles with my own eating habits and from studying Dr. Fuhrman's works. Let's take a closer look at both and then consider some solutions.

Toxic Hunger

The SAD (standard American diet) is characterized by the consumption of high-calorie, macronutrient, processed foods, oils, sweeteners, and animal products, but it's low in phytochemicals and other micronutrients. There is abundant evidence that the SAD diet results in inflammation, oxidative stress, and the accumulation of toxic waste in the body, stored in fat. These are all contributing factors to the top killers in America: cancer, heart disease, Alzheimer's and diabetes.

As a review, macronutrients are the major foods we require and eat in large amounts, mainly carbohydrates, fats, and proteins. (The problem is that we too often choose empty carbohydrates, the wrong fats, and too much protein!) Micronutrients are substances, mainly vitamins and trace minerals, which are essential in very small amounts, but are vital for healthy cell function (metabolism). These are harder to find in everyday foods. They are more readily available as phytochemicals (from plants), and they play crucial roles in human nutrition, including the optimizing of physical and mental health and the preventing and treating of various diseases. So, we're looking for quality over quantity here!

When digestion of unhealthy food is complete, the body begins to mobilize and tries to eliminate waste products (from indigestible food ingredients, excess amounts, etc.), causing uncomfortable symptoms. These sensations are symptoms of detoxification and withdrawal from an unhealthy diet that is lacking in crucial micronutrients. Scientists now know that unhealthy food has effects on the brain like those of addictive drugs. Eating healthy food does not produce drug-like withdrawal symptoms. When the body is given vegetables, fruits, beans, nuts and seeds, there is much less waste to dispose of and to detoxify from. For example, when you eat an apple, you don't feel the urge to gorge on more apples. But when you eat a chip, well... no one can eat just one.

This is why so many diets fail. Simply restricting portions of the same, unhealthy, disease-causing foods does not resolve the symptoms of toxic hunger. In addition to being effective for weight loss, I have found a nutrient-dense, plant-based diet has changed my perception of hunger, getting me in touch with true hunger. (I feel it in my throat, not in my grumbling stomach.) True hunger is a signal that directs my body to the precise number of calories needed to maintain a healthy weight. Dr. Fuhrman refers to this style of eating as a Nutritarian Diet. If widely adopted, it could bring millions of people in touch with true hunger and stop the proliferation of obesity and preventable chronic disease.

Symptoms of toxic hunger are:

- Headaches
- Weakness, shakiness and fatigue
- Stomach cramping
- Lightheadedness
- Esophageal spasms
- Growling stomach
- Irritability
- Inability to concentrate

These uncomfortable symptoms are experienced to different degrees by different individuals. The remedy for toxic hunger is to add plant-based foods back into your diet. For many of us, this needs to be done in baby steps. Upgrading your nutrition to a healthier standard needs to be a lifelong commitment, not a temporary fad diet.

Begin by adding foods that you already enjoy, then start to add foods that you don't normally eat. You'll be surprised that soon you'll be enjoying foods that you didn't like in the past. It took me three or four years to make my transition. And a big surprise to me was that I don't miss the junk food anymore and prefer healthier foods now.

Remember your body is addicted to these kinds of foods. The energy rush that is produced by the presence of high-sugar or highly processed grains creates a dopamine rush in the brain—the same phenomenon that occurs from other addictive substances like heroin! It's very hard to overcome any addiction. Here's five steps in preparing for that change:

- Remind yourself of the reasons you want to change.

- Think about your past attempts at making a change, if any. What worked? What didn't?

- Set specific, measurable goals, such as a start date, or make plans to eliminate poor nutrition choices from your life.

- Remove foods and any reminders of your addiction from your home, workplace, and other places you frequent. (Just keep walking past the donut shop!)

- Tell friends and family that you're committed to getting rid of poor nutrition, and ask for their support.

Emotional Eating

Emotional eating has been an uphill battle for me. I have a tendency to head to the fridge or the local gas station for a pick-me-up snack. If you've ever been like me and made room for dessert even though you're already full, or dove into a large bag of chips when you're feeling down, you've experienced emotional eating. Emotional eating or stress eating is using food to make yourself feel better—eating to fulfill emotional needs rather than to fill your stomach.

Using food, from time to time, as a pick-me-up, as a reward, or to celebrate isn't necessarily a bad thing, although I try to reward myself with something other than food these days. But when eating is your primary emotional coping mechanism—when your first impulse is to open the refrigerator whenever you're stressed, upset, angry, lonely, exhausted, or bored—then you get stuck in an unhealthy cycle where the underlying feelings or problems are never addressed.

Identifying Emotional Eating

Emotional hunger can't be filled with food. Eating may feel good in the moment, but the feelings that triggered the eating are still there and you often feel worse than you did before because of the unnecessary calories you consumed. You feel guilty for messing up and not having more willpower.

No matter how powerless you feel over food and your feelings, it is possible to make a positive change. You can find healthier ways to deal with your emotions, learn to eat mindfully instead of unconsciously, regain control of your weight, and finally put a stop to emotional eating.

My mom is a very loving person and an amazing cook. She grew her own garden. We had homemade meals every day when I was growing up. I think sometimes I identify eating with the love that surrounded our dinner table. So, when I am going through a hard time I naturally go to food for a loving pick-me-up. It's easy to overeat in that situation. The trick for me has been to munch on food that is highly nutritious AND filled with love—killing two birds with one stone! (Okay, not the best metaphor there!)

Signs & Symptoms of Emotional Hunger

It comes on suddenly. It hits you in an instant and feels overwhelming and urgent, usually in a time of stress, lack of sleep, or emotional pain. Physical hunger, on the other hand, comes on more gradually. For me, two triggers for eating junk food are the gas station (and the super-bad food they sell there), and junk-food advertisements. When I'm out and about, I'll bring healthy snacks along with me, and I'll look the other way when I pass a MacDonald's billboard!

It craves specific comfort foods. When you're physically hungry, almost anything sounds good—

including healthy stuff like vegetables. But emotional hunger craves junk food or sugary snacks that provide an instant rush, or remind you of a time when you ate comfort food that made you feel good. You feel like you *need* salty chips or a candy bar, and nothing else will do.

It often leads to mindless eating. Before you know it, you've eaten a whole bag of chips or an entire pint of ice cream without really paying attention or fully enjoying it. When you're eating in response to physical hunger, you're typically more aware of what you're doing.

It isn't satisfied once you're full. You keep wanting more and more, often eating until you're uncomfortably stuffed. Physical hunger, on the other hand, doesn't need to be stuffed. You feel satisfied when your stomach is full.

It isn't located in the stomach. Rather than a growling belly or a pang in your stomach, you feel your hunger as a craving that you can't get out of your head. You're focused on specific textures, tastes, and smells.

It often leads to regret, guilt, or shame. When you eat to satisfy physical hunger, you're unlikely to feel guilty or ashamed because you're simply giving your body what it needs. If you feel guilty after you eat, it's likely because you know deep down that you're not eating for nutritional reasons.

Remedies & Alternatives to Emotional Eating

1) Identify your emotional eating triggers. What situations, places, or feelings make you reach for the comfort of food? Most emotional eating is linked to unpleasant feelings, but it can also be triggered by positive emotions, such as rewarding yourself for

achieving a goal or celebrating a holiday or happy event. I had to start gassing up my truck at a different gas station because the habit and urge to go inside and buy junk food was just too overpowering for me.

2) Find other ways to feed your feelings. If you're depressed or lonely, call someone who always makes you feel better, play with your dog or cat, or go for a run to get your mind in a better frame of reference. If you're anxious, expend your nervous energy by dancing to your favorite song, squeezing a stress ball, or taking a brisk walk. If you're exhausted, treat yourself with a hot cup of tea, take a nap or go to bed early. If you're bored, read a good book, watch a comedy show, explore the outdoors, or turn to an activity you enjoy (woodworking, playing the guitar, shooting hoops).

3) Use mindful eating to press pause when cravings hit. This is a practice that develops your awareness of eating habits and allows you to pause between your triggers and your reactions.

Mindful eating helps us learn to hear what our body is telling us about hunger and satisfaction. It helps us become aware of who in the body/heart/mind complex is hungry, and how and what is best to nourish it. Mindful eating is natural, interesting, fun, and cheap. Mindful eating is eating with intention and attention. Eating is a natural, healthy, and pleasurable activity for satisfying hunger. Mindful eating is not a diet, or about giving up anything at all. It's about experiencing food more intensely—especially the pleasure of it.

Not all of these tips may feel right for you—try a few and see how they work:

- Reflect
- Sit down

- Turn off the TV (and everything else with a screen)
- Pick the smaller plate
- Skip an unhealthy item
- Serve out smaller portions
- Sprinkle with high-quality mineral salt
- Give gratitude
- Chew each bite until it's liquid before swallowing
- Savor the flavors of each item
- Put down your utensil

The bottom line that you must ask yourself: "Who's in charge here?" Both toxic hunger and emotional eating stem from OTHER factors taking over; they are NOT who you really are. It's the eating choices and habits of a lifetime run amuck. It's chemical imbalances in your brain and body from acidity and nutrient deficiency. It's the leftover emotional baggage in the subconscious from bad experiences that were not resolved in a healthy way. Are you sweeping these factors under the rug (or into ever-expanding fat cells)? Are you doing your darndest to NOT think about the obvious, impending consequences?

The truth is, YOU are in charge. You have MORE power over these factors and over your cravings than you think. Start now by planning ahead, eating consciously, feeding your body with quality not quantity, and being proactive.

You know, there's heart disease, and then there's disease in the heart. Both can kill. If you have an ache in the heart—quick, go see a doctor. If you're aching in your heart, mind, emotions and soul, that's something equally important to take a closer look at and to address. Most men are outer-directed—that's our strength, getting things done in the world—and most of us have more difficulty looking within.

That's why I put together this book FOR YOU, and why I talk about the four pillars of positive thinking, nutrition, exercise, and spirituality. Thanks for allowing this small book to be your guide. Start with small upticks in each of these four areas and you'll be very happy with the results. ☑

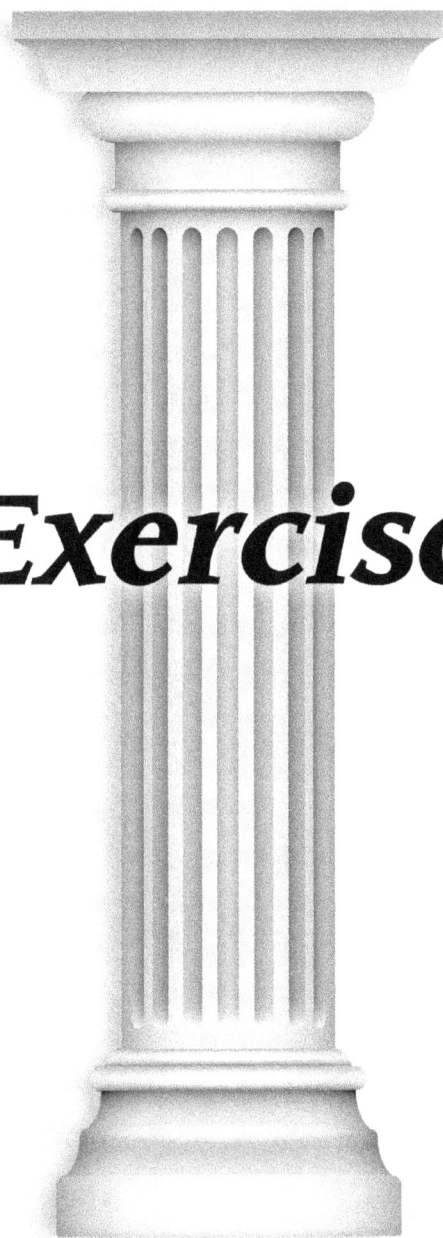

Third Pillar

Exercise

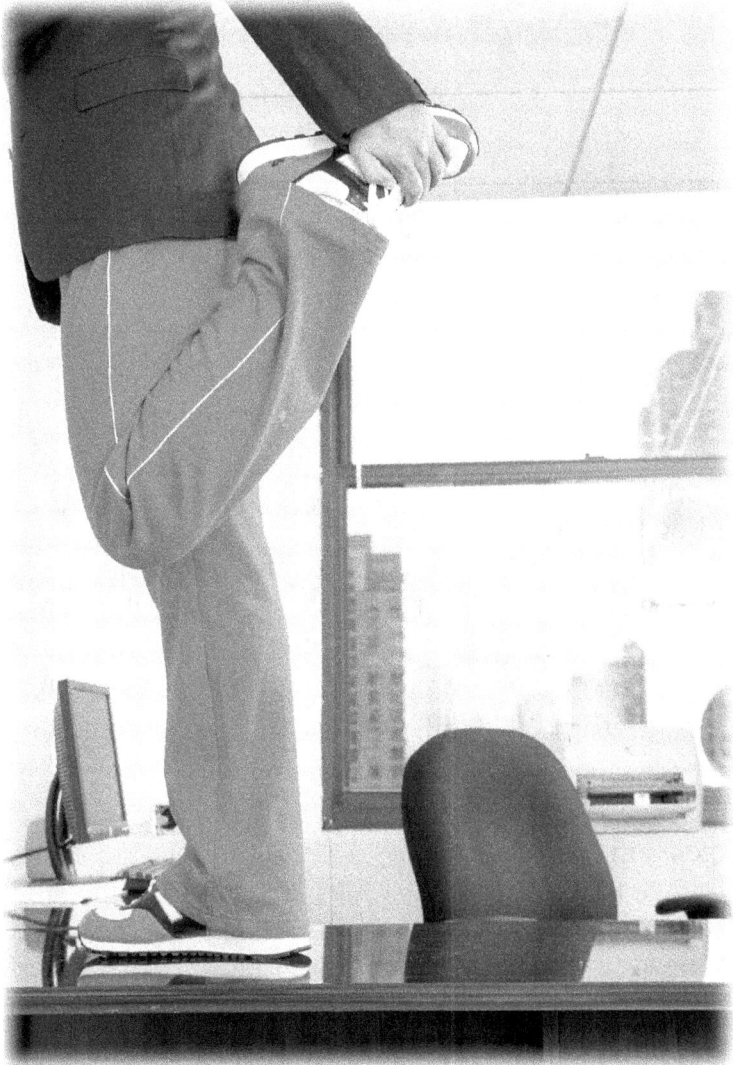

13

Getting Started

CHAPTER 13

GETTING STARTED—
Tuning Up Your Body with Exercise

To enjoy the glow of good health,
you must exercise.

—Gene Tunney,
American professional boxer
from 1915 to 1928

During high school I was a state-champion-level, long-distance runner and a wrestler. Thirty years later, things had changed. After seeing my friends suffering from diseases, and observing symptoms in my own body, I began to look for ways to get more physically active. One day I spotted a red Durasport twelve-speed bicycle at the local landfill. It looked like it worked, so I brought it home, pumped up the tires and straightened out a few things. The front brakes worked so I took it out for a spin. I went down the road about a mile and came back.

For the next two weeks, I suffered! My butt felt like someone had beaten me with a baseball bat and my leg muscles quivered every time I passed that bicycle. Not being one to give up easily, I did get back on that bike and slowly began to go farther and faster. Not too long ago I did a Century Bike Ride—130 miles over two mountain ranges—without nearly the amount of pain that I had experienced on that first two-mile ride. In this chapter I want to cover what I think exercise is, the benefits of being in shape, some tips for starting an exercise plan, what to expect of yourself, and some types of exercise you might want to check into.

A big caveat here: Please, please, please—if you are just beginning to get back into shape, get a thorough checkup from your doctor first. This is a must. Your doctor can advise you about how quickly you can jump into things and what types of exercises will be best for you. Don't side-step this or you may suffer some serious consequences.

What Is Exercise?

Exercise aims to maintain or enhance your physical fitness and general health. Do you have to ride a bike for 100+ miles? NO! Do you have to climb mountains? NO! Most of the research I've done shows that you need to get your heart pumping at an aerobic pace for 30 minutes, 3–4 times per week. Also, when you choose your exercises, mix them up so that you use as many different muscles in your body as you can. For example, in a week's time, you could mow the lawn, go swimming, do pushups, sit-ups and free weights in the garage, and go for a brisk walk with a buddy. The main thing is to be active consistently.

WHY EXERCISE?

1) Exercise controls weight

Exercise can help prevent excess weight gain and promote weight loss. When you engage in physical activity, you burn calories. The more intense the activity, the more calories you burn. Regular trips to the gym are great, but don't worry if you can't find a large chunk of time to exercise every day. To reap the benefits of exercise, simply get more active throughout your day. You can take the stairs instead of the elevator, or rev up your household chores. It's long periods of inactivity or being sedentary that seem to do the most harm to a body.

2) Exercise combats health conditions and diseases

Are you worried about heart disease, or hoping to prevent high blood pressure? No matter what your current weight, being active boosts high-density lipoprotein (HDL), the good cholesterol, and lowers high triglycerides. This one-two punch keeps your blood flowing smoothly, which decreases your risk of cardiovascular disease. Regular exercise also helps to prevent or manage a wide range of health problems including stroke, metabolic syndrome, type 2 diabetes, depression, several types of cancer, and arthritis. The increased muscle tone, balance and flexibility you'll gain can prevent falls, which have a more dangerous impact as we age.

3) Exercise improves mood

Need an emotional lift or to blow off some steam after a stressful day? A gym session or brisk, 30-minute walk can help. Physical activity stimulates various brain chemicals (endorphins) that can leave you feeling happier and more relaxed. You will probably feel better about your appearance and yourself overall when you exercise regularly, which will boost your confidence and self-esteem.

4) Exercise boosts energy

Do you get winded by walking to work, climbing the stairs, or playing with the kids? Regular physical activity can improve your muscle strength and boost your endurance. It also delivers oxygen and nutrients to your tissues and helps your cardiovascular system work more efficiently. And when your heart and lung health improves, you have more energy to tackle daily chores. It seems counter-intuitive, but our bodies are designed for activity—the more active we are, the more energy we get!

5) Exercise promotes better sleep

Regular physical activity can help you fall asleep faster and deepen your sleep. Just don't exercise too close to bedtime, or you may be too energized to get to sleep quickly.

6) Exercise puts the spark back into your sex life

Regular physical activity can increase energy levels, balance your hormones, and improve your physical appearance, which can boost your sex life. But there's even more to it than that—regular physical activity can increase your libido and your attractiveness to women. And men who exercise regularly are less likely to have problems with erectile dysfunction, compared to men who don't.

7) Exercise helps you live longer

Some researchers have found that exercise can help keep DNA healthy and young. In a small study published in the journal Science Advances, Anabelle Decottignies, from the de Duve Institute at the Catholic University of Louvain in Brussels, and her colleagues, found that just moderate-intensity physical activity helps hold back cell aging.

They studied a specific part of DNA that keeps track of how many times a cell has divided. Each time a cell divides, it copies its DNA (which is packed into chromosomes) and this section of the chromosomes, called telomeres, gets shorter. In the study, Decottignies identified a molecule that's responsible for directing this telomere-shortening, and therefore, cellular aging.

8) Exercise can be fun—and social!

Exercise and physical activity can be enjoyable. It gives you a chance to unwind, enjoy the outdoors or simply engage in activities that make you happy. Physical activity can also help you connect with family or friends in a fun social setting. Some of my most enjoyable times have been traveling to races, meets and larger events and making new friends.

Types of Exercise

There are three broad intensities of exercise:

Light—The exerciser can talk while exercising. Going for a walk and doing yard work are two examples of light exercise.

Moderate—The exerciser feels slightly out of breath during the session. Examples could be walking briskly, cycling moderately, or walking up a hill. This is aerobic exercise. Do this for 30 minutes, 3–4 times a week.

Vigorous—The exerciser is panting during the activity and is often bringing his muscles to the point of fatigue (momentary muscular failure). This could include running, cycling (indoors or out), and heavy weight training. This is a combination of aerobic and anaerobic exercise and should be done progressively and with the advice of a doctor or trainer.

The more active and the more intense your exercise (to a degree) the better your body will function and the longer it will last. Keep in mind, though, that higher-intensity workouts require longer recovery times.

TIPS FOR DEVELOPING AN EXERCISE PLAN

• Make the Time!

Start slowly. Gradually build up to at least 30 minutes

of activity, 3–4 times per week.

Exercise at the same time of day so it becomes a regular part of your lifestyle. For example, you might take a walk every Monday, Wednesday, Friday, and Sunday from noon to 12:30 p.m.

Find a convenient time and place to do activities. Try to make it a habit, but be flexible. If you miss an exercise opportunity, include some form of vigorous activity into your day in another way.

• Keep Reasonable Expectations for Yourself

If you have a high risk of coronary heart disease, or some other chronic health problem, check with your doctor before beginning a physical activity program. Start slowly with a walk around the block after dinner. Bring your wife, or walk the dog—they both will thank you!

Look for chances to be more active during the day. Walk around the mall before shopping, take the stairs instead of the escalator, or get up and be active for 10 or 15 minutes for every hour that you spend watching TV or working at the computer. Do you live in a climate with long winters, like I do? Invest in a small, indoor rebounder and keep it by your workstation. A periodic "bouncing break" boosts lymphatic drainage and immune function, increases bone mass, and improves digestion!

Don't get discouraged if you stop for a while. Get started again gradually and work up to your former improved pace. Never give up!

Don't exercise too vigorously right after meals, or when it's very hot or humid out, or when you just don't feel up to it. Remember Chapter 3: *Baby Steps—Fastest Way to the Top*?

• Make It Fun!

Choose activities that are fun and not exhausting. Add variety. Develop a repertoire of several activities that you can enjoy. That way, exercise will never seem boring or routine.

Ask family and friends to join you—you may be more likely to stick with it if you have company. Or join an exercise group, a health club or a community center. Many churches and senior centers offer exercise programs, too.

Use music or audiobooks to keep you entertained.

The past few years I have gotten involved in Triathlons. It's a sport that requires that you swim, bike and run. It's fun for me because I am not doing the same things every day. I can run one day, swim the next and bike after that. I also get a full body work out with three kinds of activities. Sticking to one thing is a struggle for me, but maybe you get a lot out of one type of activity—GREAT! HAVE FUN!

• Track and Celebrate Your Success

Note your activities on a calendar or in a logbook. Write down the distance or length of time of your activity and how you feel after each session.

Reward yourself at special milestones with non-food-splurge items, like a small gift or a shopping trip for yourself—maybe a new pair of pants that now fits you better! Nothing motivates like success.

THE BEST TYPES OF EXERCISE

If you are struggling with what types of exercises to jump into, here are four light ones that give you a full-body workout that could be fun for you. These are recommended by Dr. I-Min Lee, professor of medicine at Harvard Medical School:

1) Swimming

Many say that swimming is the perfect workout. The buoyancy of the water supports your body and takes the strain off painful joints, so you can move them more fluidly. "Swimming is good for individuals with arthritis because it's less weight-bearing," explains Dr. Lee. Research has found that swimming can also improve your mental state and put you in a better mood. Water aerobics is another, more vigorous option that helps you burn calories and tone up.

2) Tai Chi

This Chinese martial art that combines movement, breathing and relaxation is good for both body and mind. In fact, it's been called "meditation in motion." Tai Chi is made up of a series of graceful movements, one transitioning smoothly into the next. Because the classes are offered at various levels, Tai Chi is accessible and valuable for people of all ages and fitness levels. "It's particularly good for older people because balance is an important component of fitness, and balance is something we lose as we get older," says Dr. Lee. Take a class to help you get started and to learn the proper form. You can find Tai Chi programs at your local YMCA, health club, community center, or senior center. Looking for something more challenging? Yoga would be a great next step.

3) Strength Training

If you believe that strength training is a macho, brawny activity, think again. Lifting lighter weights won't necessarily bulk up your muscles, but it will keep them strong. "If you don't use muscles, they will lose their strength over time," Dr. Lee says. Increasing muscle mass also burns more calories. "The more muscle you have, the more calories you burn, so it's easier to maintain your weight," says Dr. Lee. As with other forms of exercise, strength training can also help preserve brain function in later years. Before starting a weight training program, again, be sure to learn the proper form. Start lightly, with just one or two pounds. You should be able to lift the weights 10 times with ease. After a couple of weeks, increase that by a pound or two. If you can easily lift the weights through the entire range of motion more than 12 times, you are ready move up to a slightly heavier weight.

For someone who is healthy and well into their workout routine, three sets of ten reps each, with a minute's rest in between, is considered the optimal amount per muscle group—with warm-ups, cool-downs and stretching in between.

4) Walking

Walking is simple yet powerful. It can help you stay trim, improve cholesterol levels, strengthen bones, keep blood pressure in check, lift your mood, and lower your risk for several diseases (diabetes and heart disease, for example). A number of studies have shown that walking and other physical activities can even improve memory and resist age-related memory loss. All you need is a well-fitting and supportive pair of shoes. Start with walking for about 10 to 15 minutes at a time. Over time, you can start to walk farther and faster, until you're walking for 30 to 60 minutes most days of the week.

Many of the things we do for fun (and for work) count as exercise. Raking the yard counts as physical activity. So does ballroom dancing and playing with your kids or grandkids—as long as you're doing some form of aerobic exercise for at least 30 minutes at a time. If you can include two days of strength training per week, then you can consider yourself an "active" person.

The main thing is that you get started, find a way to enjoy your exercise, and make it a lifelong habit. ☑

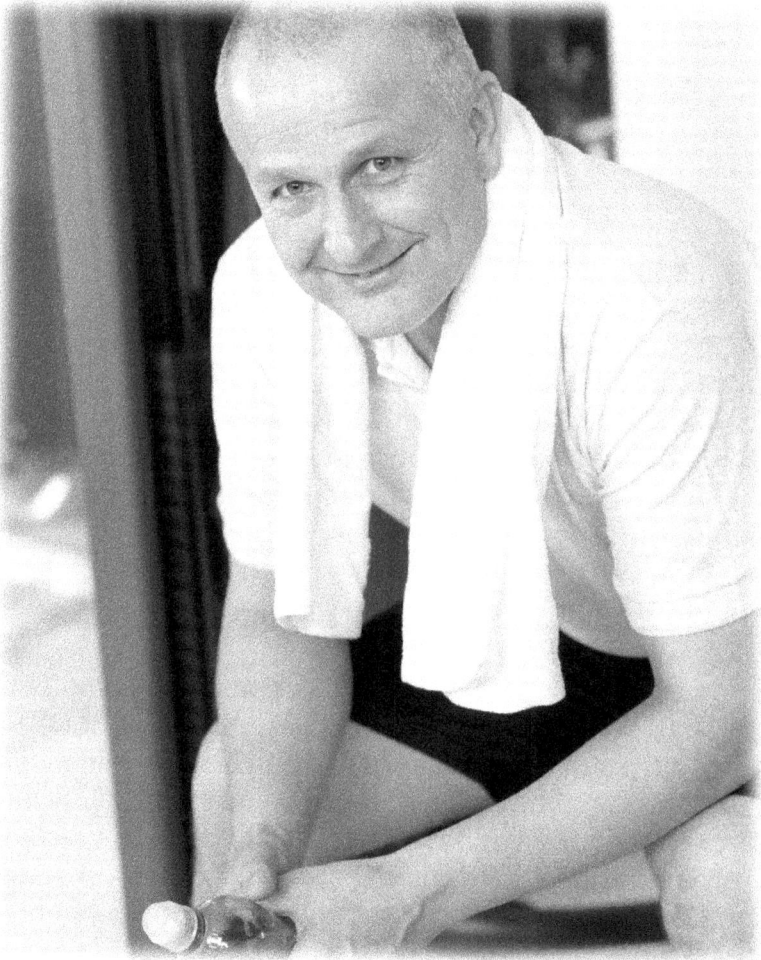

14

Exercise

CHAPTER 14

EXERCISE—
Making It a Lifestyle

*Exercise gives us an outlet for suppressed energies
created by stress and thus it tones the spirit
just as it conditions the body.*

—Arnold Schwarzenegger

Exercise? *Ugh!* It can be the most disliked word in our society. What makes it so bad? How do we stick with an exercise program? How do we turn it into a lifestyle? Here are nine strategies that I use on a consistent basis that help me build in my daily exercise as a vitally important and anticipated part of my life:

1) Commit to Regular Activity

You may not be the type of person who wants to train for a triathlon and that's perfectly okay. You don't have to become a fitness buff to benefit from exercise and movement. Start by committing to getting some form of activity into your life often during the day, especially if your work dictates that you're sitting a lot. Schedule exercise like any other appointment on your calendar and treat it as a commitment, rather than something you squeeze in only if you have time. Even if you can only allot 15 minutes at a time, schedule it. I truly believe my real fitness began when I started to use my affirmation, "I am a lean, mean machine because I eat right and exercise daily."

Take a short walk—at a leisurely pace at first, if exercise is new to you. You can build up to a power walk. If that's not your thing, take a fitness, martial arts, or yoga class, swim laps, or sign up for dance classes. Whatever exercises you start, build up slowly so you don't overwhelm yourself and then maybe give up.

2) Find your Favorite Exercise

I know people who commit to a form of exercise but they really don't like it. How long do you think they will keep that up? We aren't inclined to dive in or stick to things we despise. Out of all the forms of exercise out there, find one you just LOVE! Get specific. Don't just say, "yoga," discover what form of yoga is your favorite. If swimming is your thing, do you prefer swimming laps or doing water aerobics? Or maybe you would dread a Step class but you can't get enough of Pilates.

A good way to identify what type of exercise is right for you is to first figure out if you like to exercise alone, with a partner, or with a group or in a class. You may have to experiment a little bit before you figure that out. Try different forms of exercise until you find one that energizes you physically and mentally. Find your favorite exercise—one where excuses won't even enter the equation when it's time to exercise. And remember, there's no rule that says you must go to a gym or buy equipment. Having a variety of activities—weightlifting, walking, running, tennis, cycling, aerobics classes—will ensure that you can do *something* regardless of the weather or the time of day.

I began getting serious about staying active quite a few years ago. I have left behind relationships with people who were negative about exercising and I chose to stick with my invigorating dose of daily fitness. Friends and family members learn that it's part of your identity, and soon they give up on saying things like, "Why don't you take it easy today?"

3) Remind Yourself Daily of Your Why

It's easy to get off track if you aren't reminding yourself of WHY both working out and eating healthy are important to you. This goes back to your core motivation that we addressed. If you make it automatic to wake up and remind yourself of why exercise is important to you, you will be more likely to keep your commitments to yourself. You also will be putting exercise front and center in your day instead of treating it as an afterthought that you can skip at day's end. Wake up thinking about what exercise you will do today and it becomes a priority.

Don't get too caught up with your bathroom scale. It maybe took years for you to put on the excess weight, so give yourself some time to lose it! It's easy to get discouraged and give up when there's too much emphasis on weight loss and on seeing great results right away. Rather than an exclusive focus on weight loss, focus on how great exercise and movement make you feel instead. Take pride in your body getting stronger and in your ability to exercise longer, even if it's just in small increments. Taking the time to consider what really connects you to exercise on an emotional level is powerful because you can use those thoughts and feelings to motivate you.

Most likely, what motivates you runs much deeper than getting thinner or getting to a specific set of three numbers on a scale. Identify what that is for you. Maybe you want to have more energy for your children or grandchildren, or you want to be in more control of your health, or you want to have a lot more energy. Whatever your core motivation is, connect to that.

4) Exercising in a Group

Exercise doesn't have to be a solo endeavor. Turn it into an outing with friends and family. When you join up with others to exercise, not only do you get the immediate benefits of exercise, you also get quality time spent with friends and loved ones—a double deposit into your well-being account. When you engage in a running or bike race, you develop a sense of camaraderie and community with others.

5) Exercise Even When You're Too Tired

It's inevitable—you'll feel better after exercising. Commit to taking a first step; put on your running shoes, walk through the gym door, just take the first step. You will find taking a small step towards exercise will give you the momentum to complete your daily exercise plan.

6) Log Your Activity

Write down the things that are important to you. It could be how much time you exercise each day, how many steps you walked, how far you ran or cycled, what you weighed, etc. Some people make a game of it. You may have heard of runners calculating the miles it would take to run from their homes to Boston (home of the famous marathon), figuring how far they run in an average week, and setting a target date for "arriving" in Boston.

After your workouts, make a note of how they made you feel. This way, when you're having a particularly unmotivated day, you can look back on your accomplishments and the way exercising made you feel afterwards—endorphins will become your new BFFs—which will hopefully kick-start your motivation. It's great when your clothes fit better, when you can lift heavier weights, or work out longer without getting exhausted, but there is a slew of other progress indicators, such as:

- Getting a good night's sleep
- Less foggy thinking
- Having more energy for things you love

- Realizing your muscles aren't screaming after you've helped a friend move furniture
- Seeing your resting heart rate drop over time
- Hearing your doctor congratulate you on improved cholesterol, blood pressure, bone density, triglycerides and blood sugar levels

7) Look to the Future

Don't get caught up in guilt because you haven't been working out. Don't beat yourself up if it has been quite a while. Guilt and regret only make you feel bad; they don't get you any closer to your desired destination. With a simple decision in your mind, you can let go of what you did or didn't do and just start again. Look forward. Start over with a clear plan of what you will commit to doing each day for your health. Keep your WHY in focus.

8) Stop Comparing Yourself to Others!

It's fine to have a competitive spirit and enjoy competing with others, but what you don't want to do is start comparing yourself to others. Everyone is different and everybody achieves different things in life at different paces, plus some people are naturals in certain areas. Do your best and compete against yourself instead by trying to do just one more rep or attempting to smash your personal best time.

I just completed another half marathon and I got *passed* many times! Each time someone passed me, I had to tell myself, "Dave, run your own race. Let her pass." I got a PR (Personal Record) and was very satisfied with my run.

9) Reward Yourself

Are you telling yourself that you don't deserve a reward for something you should be doing anyway—or that once you can zip your jeans without lying on the bed, that will be reward enough? Well, honestly, how inspiring is that?

Experts say that making behavior changes is hard and that rewards motivate. So, decide on a goal and the reward you'll give yourself, and work toward it. You might buy yourself that new gadget you've wanted after you stick to your fitness plan for one month, or buy new walking shoes when you achieve 5,000 steps a day. Do whatever works for you.

Above all, believe in yourself and learn to eagerly anticipate how you will tone both your body and your spirit with your daily exercise regimen. Hopefully, these tips and tricks will help you be consistent with your personal fitness journey. I guarantee—it's worth it! ☑

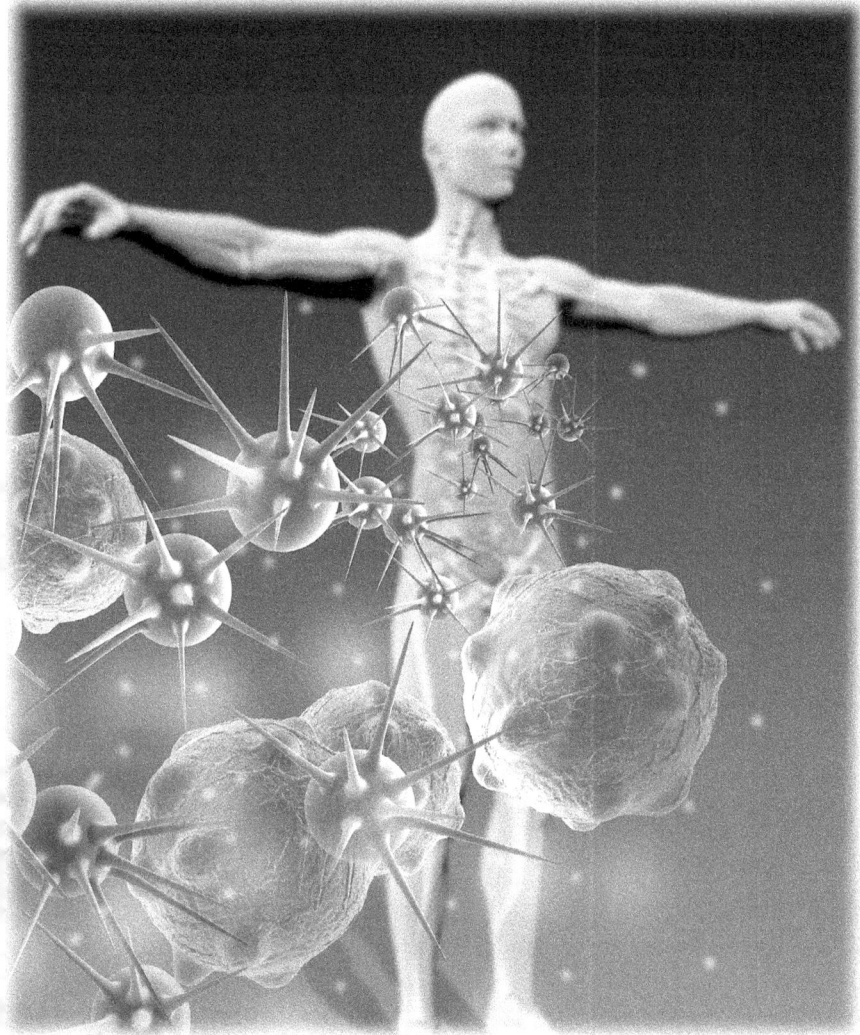

15

Our Amazing Body

CHAPTER 15

OUR AMAZING BODY—
A Self-Healing, Disease-Fighting, Strong Machine!

*If anything is sacred,
the human body is sacred.*

—Walt Whitman

One of the most amazing experiences that has happened to me as I have been focused on becoming healthy is learning how adaptable and strong my body is. I have seen my body fight diseases, grow stronger and heal itself.

A few years ago, I had a bad crash on my bike. I was cruising down the freeway at about 30 mph and hit a patch of loose gravel, causing me to tumble head-over-heels onto the side of the road. I could tell something was way wrong about my left shoulder—at 50 years old, I was afraid it might be the end of physical activity for me. I went to the hospital, got a sling, and in about 6 months I did a Century Bike Ride (100 miles).

I know the healing was sped up by my change in diet, and by giving my body the tools it needed to heal. I did visit a chiropractor to put that dislocated shoulder back in place, and then I needed two good massage sessions to calm and relax the aching and tense muscles surrounding the injury.

In addition, I have not had a cold that lasted for more than a few hours, and I have watched my body get into the best shape of my life. I am doing things today that I never dreamt of in my younger years—like going on a 28-mile trail run in the mountains behind my house in Pine Creek, a community south of Livingston, Montana.

What I hope you get out of this chapter is that you have an amazing body that can do great things if you feed it right and keep it active.

Our Bodies Can Fight Disease—The Mighty Immune System!

We have a powerful and genius immune system to help fight off all kinds of ailments. How does it work? Your immune system uses a huge army of defender cells—different types of white blood cells. You make about a billion of them every day in your bone marrow. Some of these cells, called macrophages, constantly patrol your body, destroying germs and other pathogens as soon as they are encountered. This is your natural or inborn immunity.

If an infection begins to take hold, your body fights back with an even more powerful defense of T-cells and B-cells. They give you acquired immunity, so that the same germ can never make you as ill again.

EIGHT TIPS TO STRENGTHEN YOUR IMMUNE SYSTEM

1) Food Is Medicine

You can practically double your immune system's ability to fight disease by eating more leafy greens, fruits and vegetables, and extra-nutritious superfoods. Organic fruits and vegetables are chock-full of important immune-boosting antioxidants—and they don't poison you with residues of herbicides and pesticides.

The process that is involved in the digestion of food is close to a miracle. The way the body takes raw food and converts and delivers it into hundreds of systems that your body needs to thrive is astounding and worthy of our consideration. When we put great nutrition into our body, it will use it to create a boisterous, hardworking immune system that is designed to fight off bacteria, viruses and harmful toxins.

2) Eating High-Antioxidant Foods

These are foods that fight free radicals in the body. They are one of the reasons why diseases develop and the body turns acidic instead of maintaining its alkaline balance. Free radicals have an odd (unpaired) number of electrons, so they go around robbing healthy cells to get that electron paired up. That can wreak havoc on the body. They damage the cells and cause us to age faster and to be more prone to disease. High-antioxidant foods fight free radicals because they have an extra electron to give away.

These are foods that rank high on the ORAC (Oxygen Radical Absorbance Capacity) scale. They include many herbs, like sumac, cloves and oregano. Bran, sorghum, cinnamon, turmeric, Szechuan pepper, and vanilla beans also have high ORAC values, as do many of the berries, especially blueberries and strawberries. Buy them frozen all year and use them in smoothies. (Refer to Chapter 11 on GBOMBS.)

3) Stop Eating Fast Food

Switch to raw, whole, natural, slow-absorbing foods that are better for your immune system. When you eat fast food, it most often is devoid of nutrients. And that's any processed food—if it comes in a box or a bag, it's processed! These anti-foods make your digestive system work extra hard to digest (if it can) and remove the things that give your body no benefit. If your body gets too much of these empty calories that it can't process properly, it stores the excess waste in fat cells!

There's no doubt in my mind that if I had not made the change from eating a fast-food diet to a nutrition-based diet,

I would not be able to do what I am doing today—ultra-running, Ironman, starting several new businesses, and writing this book! None of that would have happened had I continued choking down fast food. Instead, I believe by now I would be on blood-pressure medication, have achy joints and back pain, and totally lack in energy. We must quickly turn our backs on fast food!

4) Support Healthy Gut Flora

Did you know that latest research strongly links the gut microbiome (that's the "good bacteria" hidden in the walls of your digestive system) to your brain? This "brain in your gut" is revolutionizing medicine's understanding of the links between digestion, mood, overall health, and even the way you think

Eating fermented foods—yes, every day and even with every meal—is critical for gut health. The live enzymes in these foods greatly assist in the digesting of meat, especially. Foods like sauerkraut, kimchi, miso, tempeh and plain yogurt are great. Drinking either dairy or water kefir, and kombucha can greatly increase your healthy gut flora as well.

You can enjoy unsweetened dark chocolate, too, since research is showing that the beneficial bacteria that reside toward the end of the digestive tract *ferment* both the antioxidants and the fiber in cocoa.

Taking a probiotic supplement can help as well, but remember that live foods are always more powerful in what they can do for you rather than pills or capsules.

5) Get Enough Sleep

Your body can't fight free radicals and restore itself if it barely has enough energy to carry out basic functions. Make sure that when you sleep, you stay asleep soundly for 7-to-9 hours nightly. Sleeping even removes toxic waste from the body and brain! If you are having sleep problems, here are the main things you can do to improve the quality of your sleep:

a) Stick to the same bedtime and wakeup times, even on the weekends.

b) Practice a relaxing bedtime ritual, away from computers and bright lights.

c) Avoid power naps in the afternoon to make you sleepier at night.

d) Regular daily exercise greatly encourages a good night's sleep.

e) Make sure you're on a good, supportive mattress and pillow.

f) Keep any mobile phones or electric clocks far away from your bedside.

g) Sleep in a cool, dark room in order to align with your circadian rhythms.

6) Eat More Mushrooms, Onions, Garlic and Seeds

Mushrooms, onions, garlic, and seeds all have their own immune-boosting properties. Mushrooms are in the family of the "fungus-among-us" that helps to break down dead things that shouldn't be there, both in the forest and in our bodies. That is why many mushrooms are hailed as superfoods and life-enhancers in Traditional Chinese Medicine. Shiitake, rishi, and maitake are some of the best.

Onions contain fiber and folic acid, a B vitamin that helps the body make new cells. They are anti-microbial, anti-viral, and immune-boosting wonders. Eating them raw is better than cooked, because they will retain higher levels of organic sulfur compounds that provide many health benefits.

Garlic, especially when crushed or chopped and eaten raw (i.e., in salads or smoothies), may be the king of antioxidant disease-fighters. Garlic contains a compound known as allicin, which helps lower bad cholesterol and prevent blood clotting, and has anti-cancer and anti-microbial effects. Garlic is low in calories and high in nutrients, containing manganese, vitamin B6, vitamin C, selenium and fiber. Garlic protects against cell damage and aging and may also prevent, slow and even possibly reverse Alzheimer's, dementia and other brain degeneration.

Seeds are miniature plants, packed with a storehouse of all the nutrients they will need to grow big and strong, so they will do the same for you. (Remember our chapter on GBOMBS.)

7) Get Plenty of Exercise Every Day

Exercise is one of the most important ways to promote a good immune response in the body. For the best immune-boosting benefits, make walking, running, swimming, jump-roping or other sports a daily activity.

8) Whenever Possible, Use Herbs and Supplements Instead of Vaccines and Pharmaceuticals

There are many types of herbs that help boost the immune system and fight off disease. Do some research on what might work best for you. Conversely, vaccines and pharmaceuticals are extremely acidic and antibiotics can especially dampen your natural immune response and kill healthy gut flora. If your doctor insists that you need a round of antibiotics, remember to replenish your gut with fermented foods. Also, stay away from all sugary foods until your gut is back on track. Candida (yeast) will proliferate in a weakened gut, and you DON'T want to go there!

Our Bodies Can Gain Strength

Our bodies are amazing in that they can grow stronger. When I first started to get more active, my body was weak. To gain strength, I did a few things right—first I started off slowly. Second, I found activities that I enjoyed. Third, I didn't give up. By keeping after my physical conditioning, I have had doors open to me that I would not have had access to if I had given up.

So how do you strengthen muscles? You progressively overload muscles with increasingly more challenging exercises in volume, intensity, frequency or time. Then you allow the body to rest and recover, while making sure to feed it enough protein and other nutrients.

Biologically, progressive overload causes tiny tears in your muscle fibers, which your body reacts to by healing with new tissue growth, along with neurological reinforcement of recruiting those new fibers. You don't get strong by lifting the same weight repeatedly. You must push yourself harder and constantly struggle and strain to continue seeing new strength gains. You want to overload without injury, though. The key is understanding proper form, knowing your limits, and pushing hard without going too hard.

You must do a variety of exercises to strengthen different muscle groups and different ranges of motion. A gymnast has more explosive power but less endurance compared to a marathoner. A shot-putter will have a stronger upper body, while a speed-skater will have a stronger lower body, etc. They are all strong in different ways.

If you are middle aged or older, you may want to look into the benefits of super-slow weight training. It's still high-intensity and dramatically increases muscle strength, but it involves less momentum and you'll be far less likely to get injured from over-training.

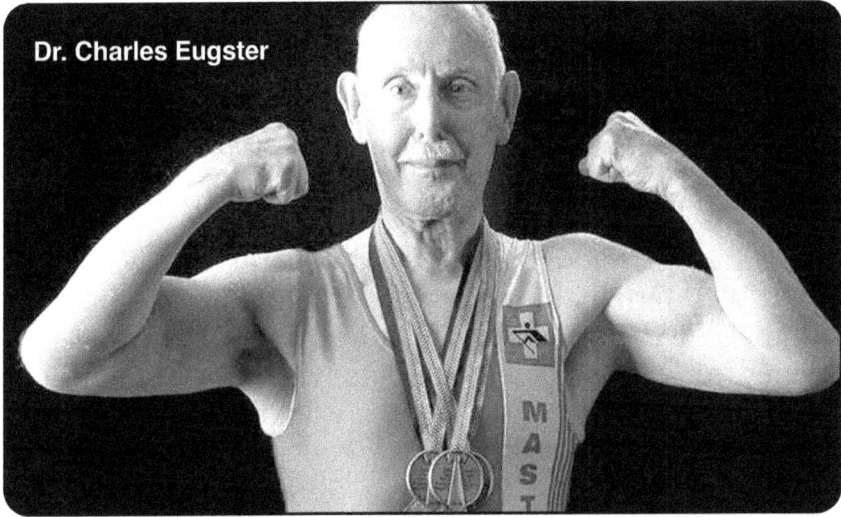

Dr. Charles Eugster

But don't sell yourself short. Dr. Charles Eugster, retired British dentist, took up bodybuilding after retiring and now, at age 96, is thought to be the world's oldest bodybuilder. He also rows and runs.

He's adamant that he's healthier and fitter now than he was in his 40s, telling the *Daily Mail*: "My ex-wife recently sent me a picture of me in my 40s and it was disgusting! I was a really horrible, self-satisfied, blobby, fat person. As a young man, I'd always been quite sporty, but I'd just let that side of things slip away... This idea that you have to wither as soon as you turn 60? Nonsense!"

And Dr. Eugster isn't the only strong older man. In 2013, great Japanese climber Yuichiro Miura became the oldest person to reach the summit of Mount Everest, at the age of 80. In June of 2015, 55-year-old US Navy veteran Rodney

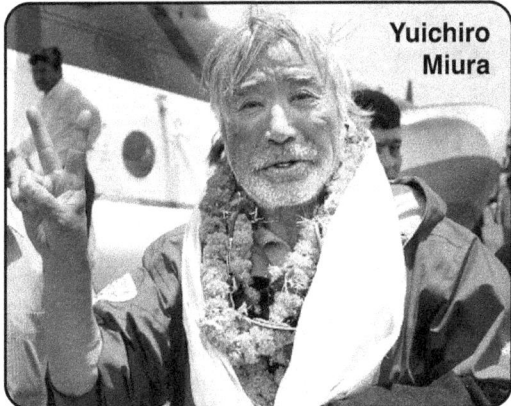

Yuichiro Miura

Hahn broke the world record for the most pull-ups (6,844) in 24 hours. The key is to start slowly and to find something you enjoy—and never give up!

The Body's Ability To Heal Itself

Stamatis Moraitis was a war veteran and was diagnosed with terminal lung cancer and told he had only six months to live. He and his wife moved into a small house on a vineyard with his elderly parents, where he reconnected with his faith and started going to his old church. Six months passed, and not only did he NOT die, he was feeling better than ever. He started making himself useful by working in the untended vineyard during the day and in the evenings, he'd play dominos with friends. At one point, 25 years after his diagnosis, Stamatis went back to ask his doctors what had happened, but the doctors had all died! He lived to be 102 years old.

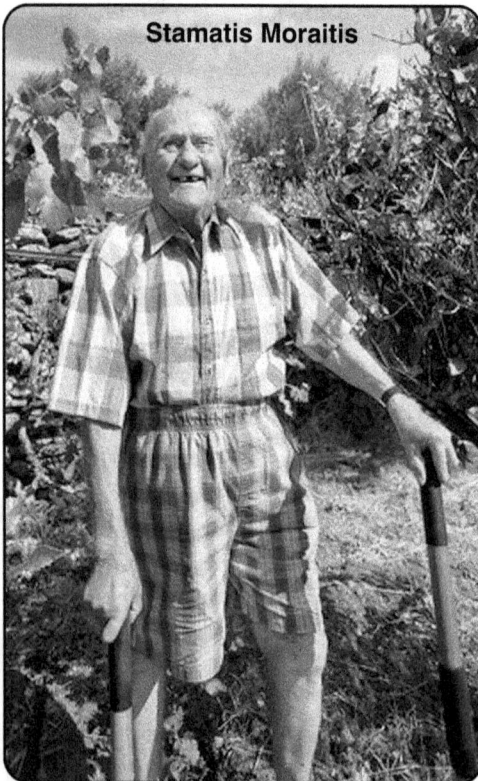

Stamatis Moraitis

The cells in your body have an amazing ability to renew themselves. In fact, all of the many trillions of cells in your entire body renew themselves every 7 to 10 years (except for the neurons in the cerebral cortex). The most fundamental unit of the human body is the cell. All human life originally begins when the sperm and ovum meet to form a single cell, which then divides into many more cells until a baby is born after nine months inside the mother's uterus.

Did you know that every second that you are alive, the cells in our bodies are endlessly working to bring us back to a natural state of homeostasis (equilibrium)? Each cell is a dynamic, living unit that is constantly monitoring and adjusting its own processes to maintain balance within the body. Cells can heal themselves, as well as make new cells that replace those that have been permanently damaged or destroyed. Even when many cells are destroyed, like on my bike wreck, the surrounding cells replicate to make new cells, thereby quickly replacing the cells that were damaged or destroyed. AMAZING!

When you have an injury where bleeding occurs in your body, blood vessels at the site contract and slow the bleeding. Next, blood platelets, which meet air, begin forming a blood clot where the injury is located. White blood cells then build up at the spot and destroy and digest dead cells by secreting special enzymes stored in small packets in the cells, called lysosomes. That way, dead-cell debris is removed and new space is made for new cells to occupy. Almost simultaneously, the process of new cell formation begins. These new cells originate mostly from the newer layers of cells of a particular tissue, while older cells are pushed to the side of the injury to gradually fill the space that was made by the injury. This amazing and complex process automatically stops when the healing is complete.

The Healing Balance of Free Radicals

A free radical is an atom that has an unbalanced pair of electrons in its outer shell, making it unstable and highly reactive. Free radicals exist within the body's cells, and they are a normal part of the process of making energy within the cell. A small percentage of the oxygen that is used to make energy goes to making free radicals. Free radicals chew up waste resulting from damage to the cell's genetic code storage (DNA). The problems begin when free radical numbers become excessive and they create disease.

Factors that increase production of free radicals in our cells include things like inflammation, infection, and extreme stress. Controlling these three should become a major focus for us as we strive for good health. More and more, people in the United States are getting wise to the fact that many diseases are avoidable, and preventing them is within our control. Whether it's the common cold, or to keep something more onerous like heart disease or cancer away, we must work at prevention and strengthening our immune function.

Help your body heal itself by getting proper sleep and rest, having a healthy diet, and getting plenty of exercise. Each of us truly oversees our body's health. And the more we work with our bodies, by giving them what they need to thrive, the less we will need to resort to prescription drugs or doctor visits.

Our bodies are so incredible! They have an impressive immune system, can grow stronger, and can heal themselves. If only we can make the right choices about nutrition, sleep and exercise—along with improving our mental outlook and thoughts, and strengthening our spiritual connection—we can all live long, active and vibrant lives. ☑

Fourth Pillar

Spirituality

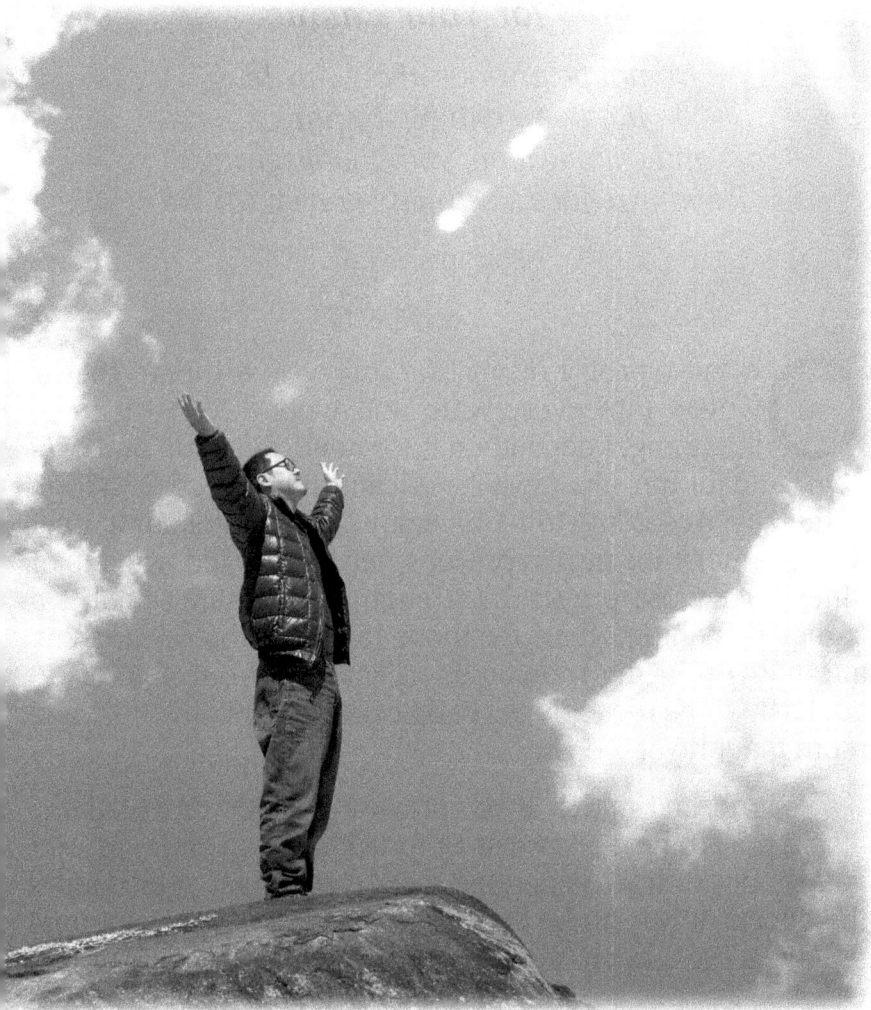

16

Prayer

CHAPTER 16

PRAYER—
Fuel for Your Engine

Do not be anxious about anything,
but in everything, by prayer
and supplication, with thanksgiving,
let your requests be made known to God.

—Philippians 4:6

On the tapestry of my life, prayer is a thread that is woven into every warp and woof. To me, it's like breathing. I depend on it for hope, direction and wisdom. And for me, like most Americans, it has become a form of therapy. According to a University of Rochester study, over 85% of Americans turn to prayer when confronted with major illness. They use prayer for strength and healing. That is a higher percentage than for those taking herbs or pursuing alternative healing modalities. (That's at about 40% of US adults by some reckonings.) People are recognizing more and more that prayer works.

It doesn't matter if you pray for yourself or for others, if you pray to heal an illness or for a change in your life, or if you simply sit in a meditative silence and quiet your mind— the effects appear to be the same. A wide variety of spiritual practices have been shown to alleviate the stresses of life, which are one of the major contributing factors for the onset of disease. Any spiritual practice is also a powerful way to maintain a positive outlook and successfully weather the trials that come to all in life.

The relationship between prayer and health has been the subject of scores of double-blind studies over the past four decades. Dr. Herbert Benson, a cardiovascular specialist at

Harvard Medical School and a pioneer in the field of mind/body medicine, discovered what he calls "the relaxation response" that occurs during periods of prayer and meditation. I believe and have every confidence that men who pray are healthier.

FOUR IMPORTANT REASONS TO PRAY

1) It Makes Us Healthier

Physiological changes occur when we pray. The body's stress response decreases, the heart rate slows, blood pressure goes down, and our breath becomes calmer and more regular, putting us in a healthier place and bolstering the immune system.

2) It Builds Relationship

Communication is the lifeblood of any relationship and it's the same in our relationship with God. It is the great desire of God's heart to have a personal relationship with YOU! We were created for an intimate relationship with God—it's built in—and prayer is our vital role in that relationship.

3) It Makes a Difference

Imagine that someone in your family has an illness for which the doctor prescribes several types of medication. He or she receives the medicines—and then upon arriving home, only takes one of the medicines prescribed. That would be crazy, wouldn't it? God, the Master Physician, the All-Knowing, our Loving Father, has given us prayer to assist in times of need. If prayer is prescribed to us by God—as a means of releasing His grace and power into situations—why would we NOT participate in it? Why would we hold back the benefits of prayer and make that critical difference for ourselves and others?

I was a children's pastor for seven years. A vivid memory I have of that time is when I set forth to help the kids understand that prayer really does make a difference. We decided to do a "test." For eight weeks, we would begin our children's church program with prayer and kids would raise their hands and submit prayer requests. Our secretary would record them. The next week, we would do the same thing except that we would read the list from the previous week. I thought it would be good for the kids to see many of their prayers answered over time.

I had no idea that the results would be so astonishing! By the end of the eight-week trial, more than 90% of the prayers had been answered and almost all of them were answered in the way the kids had requested. I have often thought it would be a good idea for me to do that for myself and family on an ongoing basis. I bet I would be surprised once again.

4) It Fulfills Our Destiny

The Lord's Prayer says: *Your Kingdom come, Your Will be done, on Earth as it is in Heaven.* [Matthew 6:10] Prayer is not just for times of need. Jesus instructed us to pray always for God's Will and purposes to be accomplished through us. God's Will for us can only be known; our destiny can only be fulfilled as fruit of that communion.

SIX BENEFITS OF PRAYER

1) Connects Us to the Spiritual World

Remember the TV show *The Twilight Zone*? It was a show about entering alternate universes. Something like that happens when we pray—you cross over into the higher realms where God and the angels dwell, you connect with that mysterious spiritual world and have access to the power that's there for the asking.

2) Improves Self-Control

Studies have demonstrated that self-control is like a muscle and the research indicates that prayer can help you strengthen your "self-control muscle." Research participants who said a prayer prior to a mentally exhausting task were better able to exercise self-control following that task. In addition, other studies demonstrate that prayer reduces alcohol consumption, reflecting the exercise of self-control. (Ask anyone in AA about that.) Findings such as these suggest that prayer has an energizing and empowering effect.

3) Increases Calm and Well-Being

Remember the guy who cut you off on the freeway? Remember the rage you felt? Why do we respond that way? Researchers found that having people pray for those in need reduced the aggression they expressed following an anger-inducing experience. In other words, prayer helps you NOT lose your cool. Next time that guy cuts you off, try praying for him— he probably needs it!

4) Makes You More Forgiving

Researchers found that when people prayed about a situation with a romantic partner or a difficult friend, it made them able to empathize with and be more willing to forgive those individuals. When we pray to God, who loves us in spite of our "issues," it helps us cut some slack to people around us. When we realize how much unconditional love and understanding we've received from our Heavenly Father, it's easier to pass that along to others.

5) Increases Trust

Recent studies found that having people pray together with a close friend increased feelings of unity and trust. This finding is interesting because it suggests that praying with others can be an experience that brings people closer together. Social prayer may thus help build close relationships. *For where two or three are gathered together in my name, there am I in the midst of them.* [Matthew 18:20]

6) Offsets the Negative Effects of Stress

Researchers found that people who prayed for others were less vulnerable to the negative physical effects associated with financial and other stresses. It was the focus on others that seemed to be contributing to the stress-buffering effects of prayer. However, praying for material gain did not counter the effects of stress. So being concerned about the welfare of others seems to be a crucial component of receiving personal benefits from prayer.

HOW TO PRAY

But, you may ask, what is the proper way to pray? Saint Paul, in Philippians 4:6-7 instructs us to pray without being anxious, to pray about everything, and to pray with thankful hearts. God will answer all such prayers with the gift of His peace in our hearts. The proper way to pray is to pour out our hearts to God, being honest and open with God, as He already knows us better than we know ourselves. We are to present our requests to God, keeping in mind that God knows what is best and will not grant a request that is not His will for us.

Even Jesus, in the Garden of Gethsemane before his final trials, prayed with these words: *Father, if thou art willing, remove this cup from me; nevertheless, not my will, but thine be done!* [Luke 22:42] We are to express our love, gratitude, and worship to God in prayer without worrying about having just the right words to say. God is more interested in the content of our hearts than the eloquence of our words.

Jesus gave a pattern for prayer, *The Lord's Prayer,* in Matthew 6:9-13. This is an example of the things that should go into a prayer—worship, trust in God, requests, confession, and submission. Praying for the things that *The Lord's Prayer* talks about, using our own words and customizing it to our own journey with God, is the way to tune into the spiritual world and connect with God. Be careful about the rote repetition of ANY prayer, without fully engaging your heart and mind. God's desire is for prayer to be a real and personal connection between Himself and us.

As someone recently put it: "We are not human beings having a spiritual experience—we are spiritual beings having a human experience!" Prayer opens up doorways that can be opened in no other way. Spending time in prayer has many benefits that we can feel the results of right away. And who knows how one prayer will reverberate and have its effects throughout both this world and the next before its blessings return to us multiplied? ☑

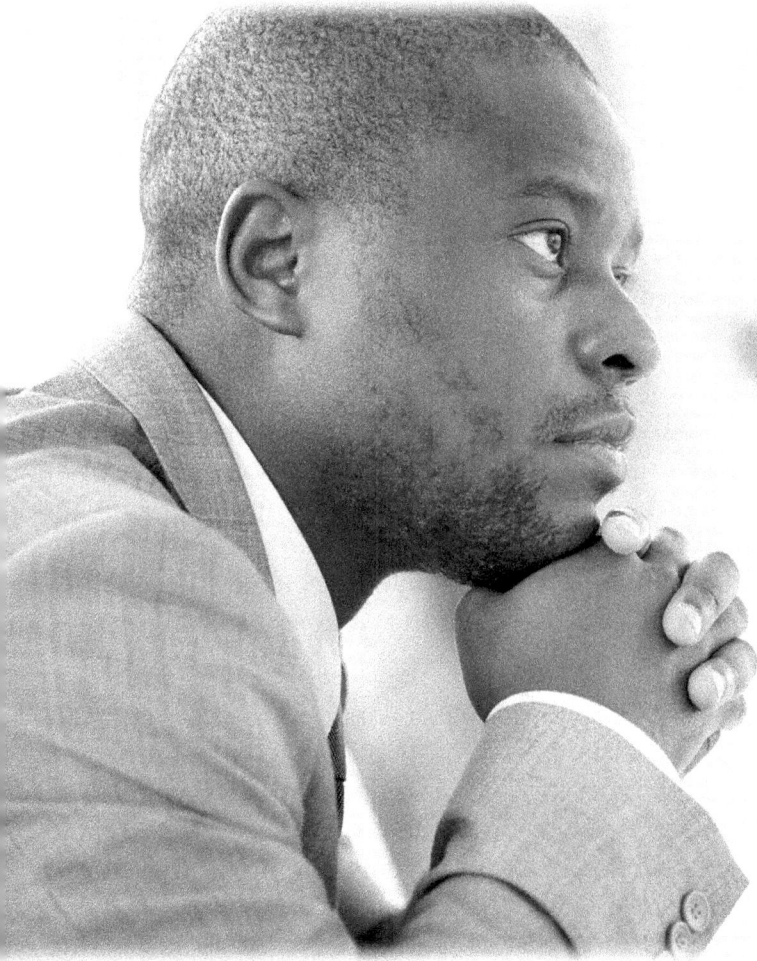

17

Meditation

CHAPTER 17

MEDITATION—
A Power Tool for the Mind & Spirit

At the end of the day, I can end up just totally wacky,
because I've made mountains out of molehills.
With meditation, I can keep them as molehills.

—Ringo Starr, British singer and songwriter,
drummer for the Beatles

Some of the most transformative moments of my life have been when I was in a state of meditation and became enlightened as to a direction or a situation in my life. It's a time when I let go of my own agenda, fears and limitations and seek guidance from God and the scriptures. In contrast to prayer when I am actively engaged in communication with my Creator, meditation is a time of just being quiet and listening.

I remember long walks on dark roads as I contemplated a dark situation I was in, getting reassurance and hope that things would be okay. It was a hard time in my life. I had been in business for myself remodeling a house and had made plenty of mistakes. I was faced with a $150,000 bill from the IRS that I had no way of paying. A family member was facing serious medical issues. The economy was in a slump. I couldn't sleep, common for me in those days, so I went out walking down that dark road at 3 o'clock in the morning. I was out of ideas and desperate.

As a last resort I did the only thing I had left—I turned to God and asked for help. In humility and great release, I remember thinking, "I am finished. I have destroyed my family. We're going to lose our home and all our dreams. Please God, HELP!"

I don't know how long I walked that night, but I remember thinking about how God had helped us in the past and reflecting on some personal spiritual experiences that I had in the past. It wasn't long before I started to feel hopeful and went back to my house. We did make it through that time with our finances intact. We were able to remodel that house and made a good profit. I think if it weren't for that time of meditation I would have lost all hope.

Many times, meditation has helped me refocus and re-energize on the important things in my life. I also remember sunshiny times and gentle breezes after climbing to a mountaintop, when I would feel an overwhelming sense of gratitude and joy. I now take some time each time I am in the mountains to just sit and enjoy the place—just being in the moment and feeling everything intensely that comes to my senses: the sights, the smells, the sounds, the tastes, and the majesty of the location. It all adds up to the feeling of a powerful presence around me that I would not have experienced if I had not taken the time to meditate.

When I think of meditation, I think of three things—silence, stillness and simplicity. Silence means letting go of thoughts. Stillness means letting go of desires. Simplicity means letting go of self-analysis.

You can meditate multiple times a day, every day. This daily practice may take some time to grow into, and admittedly, I struggle to be consistent with it myself. But be patient. Remember what we learned in Chapter 3—take baby steps. When you give up or get discouraged with your inability to quiet your mind, start again.

Check out what's going on in your community. You may find that a meditation group and a connection with community may help you to develop this discipline. It's a discipline rather than a technique. Start taking some steps. Soon it will get ingrained in your life. Experience is the best teacher. It allows the benefits and fruits of meditation to pervade your mind and all aspects of your life. Catholic priest John Main said that, "Meditation verifies the truths of your faith in your own experience."

I meditate to take the attention off my various outer selves, seeking guidance from God. In the Christian tradition, contemplation is a grace and is a reciprocal work of love. Not surprisingly, then, if we find we become more loving people because of meditating this will express itself in all our relationships, in our work, and in our sense of service, especially to those in need.

You are going to reap a whole lot of benefits when you make meditation a part of your lifestyle. This is what I have experienced. Let's go over some of them:

Your faith will increase, since this is your chance to develop a stronger connection with God. Expect that your relationships will improve. You will have much more faith in God and yourself.

You will learn to love God more. You will be aware of the things he has done for you. This will allow you to enjoy the smallest and simplest blessings that come your way.

You will be more apt to be free from worry and stress. As you grow in meditation, you will have less on your mind that will cause anxiety or pain. Enjoying a healthy and fun-filled life is what meditation provides you with.

You will understand the meaning of the passages in the scriptures, along with the plan and purpose that Christ has for you!

Here are 9 of my favorite things to do mindfully and in preparation for meditation:

1) Listening to inspirational music

Sing along, and feel your body vibrate with the hum of sound. Listen carefully to each word and each instrument.

2. Drinking tea, coffee, or a smoothie

I imagine that, like me, you drink something every morning. Instead of just tossing it down in a big gulp, drink it slowly. Dedicate 5–10 minutes every morning to this act alone. Close your eyes, and feel the liquid roll over your tongue. Enjoy it—and be silent and still!

3. Swimming

Swimming can be a long, tedious experience at times. Sometimes, I memorize a scripture or important phrase and mull it over in the pool or lake while I am swimming.

4. Driving to work

I drive a lot. You might have a daily commute. This time can be spent in absolute mindfulness. Turn off the loud music, tone down your road rage, and enjoy the quiet time to yourself.

5. Taking a walk

A slow one, as in really slow! Inhale and lift your foot, exhale and plant it. Repeat.

6. Writing in a journal each morning

Spill out a page of junk that's been on your mind. Notice the pressure of the pen on the paper, the sound of the tip scraping along the page, and the way the ink bleeds. After writing for a bit about your day, and your to-do list, and the next big project on the horizon, you'll find that you don't have anything left to write. This is when you take a deep breath, and allow mindfulness to permeate. Go deeper. Soon, you'll be writing with complete presence, as if another voice is writing through you.

7. Biking

Getting on my bike with some contemplative worship music playing in my earbuds creates an extremely peaceful time for me.

8. Eating

Not only is eating mindfully a simple and delightful act, but it's much healthier than shoveling food down while you're running to your next meeting or while watching some mindless show on TV. Take time to feel the temperature of your food with your fingers, feel the texture, and smell all the ingredients. Be there with your food before you eat and bless it before you begin. Be still and silent.

9. Breathing

The easiest of all! Breathing truly is the difference between feeling anxious and feeling relaxed. The following exercise slows down your autonomic nervous system from "fight-or-flight" to "rest, digest and heal" in no time... Try adding ten rounds of breathing with a 4, 4, 8 count into your daily routine. Inhale for 4 counts (be sure your belly and lower torso expands, rather than doing a high-chest breath), hold your breath for 4 counts, and then exhale more slowly for 8 counts. Close your eyes. Repeat for at least ten cycles. Then be still and silent.

Things are so fast-paced these days. I don't think we were designed for full-speed-ahead all the time. Taking time to meditate gives us an opportunity to slow down and to refocus and re-energize on the most important aspects of our lives. There are vitally important perceptions that can happen, but only when we be still and silent and keep it simple. ☑

Be still, and know that I am God:
I will be exalted among the nations,
I will be exalted in the earth.

—Psalm 46:10

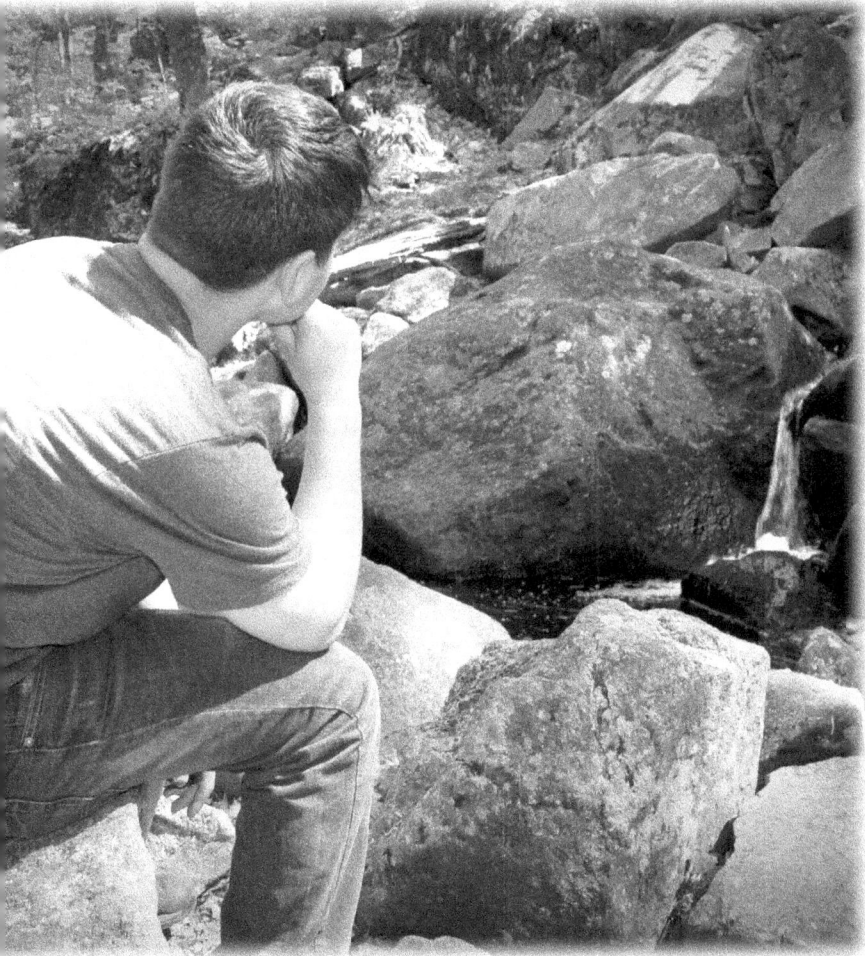

18

Fasting

CHAPTER 18

FASTING—
Ninja Health

*Instead of using medicine,
rather, fast a day.*

—Plutarch,
Greek biographer and essayist

During my fasts, I have had some of the most amazing experiences of my life. Physically—I found that I am more disciplined than I ever thought I could be, and that my body could do things I never imagined. Mentally—I received clarity of thought and rest from a chattering mind. I felt like I was in an altered state during my fasts. Emotionally—I experienced emotions I didn't know I had, both good and bad. Spiritually—I got tuned into my Creator in a way that was so real and dynamic, words can't describe it.

I was interested in taking my health and spiritual life to a new level. I started with a one-day fast, then moved to a three-day fast, and progressed from there. The longest fast I have done was 18 days. Please do some research and consult your physician to make sure a fast is right for you. I found Dr. Joel Fuhrman's *Fasting and Eating for Health* quite helpful as a guide.

Each time I fasted, it was different—a hard but rewarding experience. I had strong emotional swings—in both directions. One time at about day 12, I was relaxing in a local hot-springs pool when a kid walked by me with a burger and fries on a plate. It was like an inner monster raged up from inside me with a strong desire for that food. It was almost uncontrollable, like Gollum, the devious character in Tolkien's *Lord of the Rings*, who desired the ring of great power. That emotion of hunger for the food and even jealousy and anger toward the innocent kid took me off guard and came from a dark spot inside of me that I had to observe, and obviously, not act upon. Perhaps it was the survival instinct, like the hungry stray dog wanting to pounce on a meaty bone—the hamburger, not the kid!

I felt like this point in my fasting was a time of deep release for me, as those emotions were exposed and dealt with in a healthy way. In the positive direction, I also experienced times of inner peace and spiritual elation that were wonderful and life-changing, with a clear mind and a pain-free and like-new energized body.

At some point, I would like to do a 30-day fast because I don't think I completed all the work I needed to get done in 18 days. During each of the fasts I do, I drink only water, no food. Some people believe that you should fast for shorter periods but more frequently and on a consistent basis, like one day a week. Although I haven't tried this, I can see how it would be of value for good health.

In this chapter, you will learn how your body reacts when you stop feeding it. We'll look at 11 benefits of fasting, and we'll summarize the stages you go through as you proceed along an extended fast.

How your Body Reacts When You Stop Eating

When you eat, your digestive system breaks down carbohydrates into the sugar, glucose, which is the body's major source of energy. Glucose is absorbed from the digestive tract into the blood and then travels to your body's cells to provide them with fuel.

If you haven't eaten recently, the supply of glucose in your blood drops and your body turns to stored glucose, called glycogen, for energy. Once the glycogen is used up, your body begins to burn fat (first) and muscle (as a last resort) to make its own glucose to fuel your cells.

After a few days without eating your body kicks into ketosis mode, which some experts advise against, while others highly recommend. Ketosis is the bodily state where you burn fat as the primary source of fuel to spare muscle. You will lose weight in the form of lost body fat. However, ketosis also makes your blood more acidic (the result of shedding excess toxins stored in body fat), and can cause bad breath, fatigue, and other unpleasant but short-term symptoms. Long-term fasting, some experts warn, can lead to kidney and liver damage.

Like beginning an exercise regimen, you should only consider fasting under the supervision of a health-care professional. When counseling a friend recently who was about to go on a fast, he related his experience of seeking advice at the local clinic and hospital. The personnel there advised him against fasting altogether, which is a typical response from those in traditional Western medicine.

Perhaps they are forgetting the biblical perspective of Jesus' fasting for 40 days and 40 nights in preparation for his greatest mission. I recommended that my friend go to see a naturopathic physician for blood work and a check-up prior to his fasting and for additional guidance and supervision.

My thoughts on fasting and losing weight are that it is generally not a good idea to fast to lose weight. Number one, it's not always a permanent solution. Although I did lose weight during my fast, within two months I had gained it all back. Number two, healthy weight loss is done by choosing healthy nutrition and dealing with toxic hunger and emotional eating. Check out Chapter 12 for an in-depth look at these issues. While fasting can temporarily take away one's cravings, if the emotional and mental issues behind them are not dealt with, they will probably come back.

BENEFITS OF FASTING

1) Promotes Detoxification

The practice of abstaining from processed foods filled with additives, refined sugars, and acidic, hard-to-digest animal proteins, even for a short period of time, allows the body to begin cleansing the debris built up in the lymphatic and digestive systems. Because excess toxins that the body can't deal with at the time are stored in fat and the body uses up fat for energy during fasting, especially after 3 or 4 days, fasting can be very beneficial for cleansing, detoxifying and self-healing.

2) Rests the Digestive System

During a fast, the digestive organs rest. The normal physiological functions continue, but at a reduced rate. Because the digestive process is constantly bombarded by food to break down, an opportunity to rest reduces the energy expenditure sent to those organs, and instead can go to areas of the body that need more attention and healing. By abstaining from acidic food options (meat, dairy products, refined grains, sugar, alcohol and coffee), the production of stomach acid also reduces, hence many experience relief from ulcers during their fasting period.

3) Resolves Inflammatory Response

Some studies show that fasting promotes resolution from inflammatory diseases and allergies, including rheumatoid arthritis, joint pain and skin issues. The obvious cause of this relief is that inflammation-producing foods have stopped being consumed, therefore the body can flush out acid waste, the main cause of inflammation, and heal itself.

4) Reduces Blood Sugar

Fasting increases the breakdown of glucose so that the body can get energy, which in effect reduces the production of insulin and rests the pancreas. Glucagon is produced to facilitate the breakdown of glucose; therefore, the outcome of fasting is a reduction in blood sugar.

5) Promotes a Healthy Diet

It has been observed that fasting reduces craving for processed foods and promotes a desire for natural, water-rich foods such as fruits and vegetables. A healthy lifestyle is imperative to maintain optimum nourishment and health, therefore fasting is one way of jump-starting detoxification, stopping cravings, and adopting a healthier diet.

6) Boosts Immunity

When an individual is on a balanced diet in between fasts, this can boost immunity. Elimination of toxins and reduction in fat stores also helps the body. When intelligently breaking a fast with fruit, one can increase the body's stores of essential vitamins and minerals, such as Vitamin A and E, which are great antioxidants readily available in fresh produce. Consuming a wide range of phytonutrients helps to boost immunity.

7) Helps Overcome Addictions

According to many sources, fasting makes it easier to kick the habit, whether with alcohol, nicotine, sugary-food or refined-flour consumption. With any addiction, once your body starts to detoxify from the substance, you will crave it and experience dramatic detox symptoms until stores are replenished, or until you complete the detox process. Abstaining from addiction triggers while fasting allows the body to detoxify those acids and toxins from the bloodstream and cells, and can help you stop those cravings for good.

Highly mineralizing and alkalizing green leafy vegetables have been shown to be exceptionally beneficial for reducing cravings as part of a healthy diet. Ramp them up in your diet once you break your fast.

8) Corrects High Blood Pressure

Aside from adopting a healthier diet, fasting is one of the non-drug methods of reducing blood pressure. It helps to reduce the risk of atherosclerosis, which is the clogging of arteries by fat particles (associated with eating a highly refined, high-animal-protein diet with inflammation-promoting chemicals and additives).

Since glucose and later, fat stores, are used to produce energy during fasting, metabolic rate is reduced during fasting and the fight-or-flight hormones such as adrenaline and noradrenaline are also reduced. These all work together to keep the metabolism steady and within limits, the effect of which is a reduction in blood pressure.

9) Spiritual Benefits

Many of us think of fasting as a spiritual duty to God, depriving ourselves of food and drink for a period of time in order to prove our love for Him. While long-suffering is a part of being human and certainly a part of being a Christian, fasting should not be included when we think about "suffering for Christ."

On the contrary, fasting is less about what we're giving up and much more about what we're making room for. When we fast, we exchange what we need to survive on and make room for what we need to thrive on—more of God. Here are five spiritual benefits to fasting that I've experienced:

a) **A soul cleansing.** Without the toxins we put into our bodies, we not only give our bodies a break from the digestive process, but we also allow our spirits to be detoxed. By fasting, we cleanse the soul and make it new so we can receive the Holy Spirit and become empowered to live for Christ in a new way.

b) **A new desire for God.** When we realize we need God more than we need food, we can start to understand what the Psalmist meant when he wrote, "Like the deer that pants after water, my soul longs for You."

c) **A deeper praise.** Because the body does not have to do the work of digestion, it has more energy to focus on other things. We'll be celebrating the things of the Spirit the whole time without being distracted by food!

d) **A sensitivity to God's voice.** When we detox our spirit, and become consumed with desire and praise for God, we become sensitive to His voice. When our fasting is done, and God speaks to us in the midst of chaos, we'll still be able to pick out His voice and know what He wants us to do because we have trained our ear to hear Him through fasting.

e) **A new satisfaction.** When you finish your fast, renewed and full of energy, detoxed and with a new desire, a new praise, and a new sensitivity to God's voice, you'll find that the absence of food was small in comparison to what you gained.

Physical food never fully satisfies. In a few hours, you'll need to eat again. But when you are filled from doing the work of the Lord, you will find a new satisfaction like you've never experienced.

STAGES OF FASTING

STAGE 1: Days 1 & 2

On the first day of fasting, the blood-sugar level drops below 70 mg/dl. To restore the blood to the normal glucose level, liver glycogen is converted to glucose and released into the blood. This reserve is enough for about half a day. The body then reduces the basal metabolic rate (BMR). The rate of internal chemical activity in resting tissue is lowered to conserve energy. The heart slows and blood pressure is reduced. Glycogen is pulled from the muscle causing some weakness.

The first wave of cleansing is usually the worst. Headaches, dizziness, nausea, bad breath, glazed eyes and a heavily-coated tongue are signs of the first stage of cleansing. Hunger can be the most intense in this period unless an enema or colon hydrotherapy is used, which quickly assists the body into the fasting state by ending digestion in the colon.

STAGE 2: Days 3 to 7

Fats, composed of transformed fatty acids, are broken down to release glycerol from the molecules and converted to glucose. The skin may become oily as rancid oils are purged from the body. People with problem-free skin may have a few days of skin eruptions. A pallid complexion is also a sign of waste in the blood. Ketones are formed by the incomplete oxidation of fats. The ketones in the blood are said to suppress the appetite by affecting the food-satiety center in the hypothalamus. You may feel hungry for the first few days of the fast, but the effect is temporary—the desire to eat will subside. Lack of hunger may last from 40 to 60 days, depending on whether you are on water, a green drink, or juice.

The body embraces the fast and the digestive system can take a much-needed rest, focusing all its energies on cleansing and healing. White blood cell and immune system activity increases. You may feel pain in your lungs. The cleansing organs and the lungs are in the process of being repaired. Periodically, the lymphatic system expels mucoid matter through the nose or throat. The volume excreted of this yellow-colored mucus can be large. The sinuses go through periods of being clogged, then will totally clear. The breath is still foul and the tongue coated. Within the intestine, the colon is being repaired and impacted feces on the intestinal wall start to loosen.

STAGE 3: Days 8 to 15

On the latter part of an extended fast, after the first week, you can experience enhanced energy, clear-mindedness and feel better than you have since childhood. On the downside, old injuries may become irritated and painful. This is a result of the body's increased ability to heal during fasting. If you had broken your arm 10 years before, there is scar tissue around the break. At the time of the break, the body's ability to heal was directly related to lifestyle. If you lived on a junk-food diet, the body's natural healing ability was compromised.

During fasting, the body's healing process is at optimum efficiency. As the body scours for dead or damaged tissue, the lymphocytes enter the older, damaged tissue, secreting substances to dissolve the damaged cells. These substances irritate the nerves in the surrounding region and cause a reoccurrence of aches from previously injured areas that may have disappeared years earlier. This pain is a good sign, as the body is completing an overdue healing process. The muscles may become tight and sore due to toxin irritation. The legs can be the worst affected, as due to gravity, toxins accumulate in the legs and feet. Cankers are common in this stage due to the excessive bacteria in the mouth. Daily gargling with salt water will prevent or heal cankers.

STAGE 4: Days 16 to 30

The body is completely adapted to the fasting process. There is more energy and clarity of mind. Cleansing periods can be short with many days of feeling good in between. There are days when the tongue is pink and the breath is fresh. The healing work of the organs is being completed. After the detoxification mechanisms have removed the causative agents or rendered them harmless, the body works at maximum capacity in tissue proliferation to replace damaged tissue.

While a short fast will reduce the symptoms, a longer fast can completely heal the body. Homeostatic balance is at optimum levels. The lymphatic system is running clean except for a rare discharge of mucus through the nose or throat. After day 20, the mind is affected. Heightened clarity and emotional balance are felt at this time. Memory and concentration improve.

STAGE 5: Breaking the Fast

It's critical after extended fasting to ease back into food slowly and purposefully. Start with sips of fruit juice to get your digestive system back in good working order. If you desire something warm, a vegetable broth, no meat yet, is ideal.

Don't cram a bunch of heavy food into your system right after a fast. Don't give yourself permission to binge on low-nutrient, high-calorie food as a reward after a fast. You'll be sorry if you do because your system won't react well and it will take days to recover.

Toxins enter the blood through a congested colon. The gallbladder dumps its waste in a heavy discharge of bile. After a good fast, the sticky, toxic, mucoid coating on the intestinal wall is loose, and the first meal frees it from the intestinal wall. Eating a high-fiber fruit, like an apple or berries, with plenty of chewing, can help this sweeping-out process. This can cause an instant bowel movement upon eating, followed by intense diarrhea.

Hold off on meat and dairy for several days. Introduce a small number of nuts and beans first, after a few days of fruits and vegetables. Your stomach has shrunk, so you won't want much food.

[These *Fasting Stages* were adapted from the online forums at CureZone.org.]

FASTING VARIATIONS

There are several modifications on the strict water fast that deserve to be explored here. Abstinence is when you remove certain harmful foods from your diet for a period of time, such as with vegetarianism (no meat, poultry or seafood) and veganism (avoiding all animal products including dairy, eggs and honey). These are abstinences from which people all around the world, for centuries, have found benefits. And again, even a temporary or occasional respite from harmful or junk foods will be of benefit.

There is mono-eating—a meal consisting of just one food, which gives the body a rest from digesting a vast array of food combinations. And there is mono-fasting, such as the brown-rice fast that many recommend. The fiber in the rice produces a scrubbing action on the digestive tract. Lengthy fruit fasting, because of fruit's high-sugar content, is now less recommended, for that reason.

A superfood fast is probably the easiest and safest way to fast. A superfood is a plant-based (single or in combination) food supplement that contains a high concentration of vitamins, minerals, omega fatty acids and amino acids—just-about everything the body needs in terms of nutrition—but the catch is that superfoods are very low in calories. Some are as low as 30 calories per serving. This would reduce your typical calorie intake from 2,000–3,000 per day to as low as 90 per day (3 servings of a superfood and water). Your body remains well nourished, thus reducing some of the starvation symptoms of fasting, yet the body still goes into ketosis and burns fat. (Note: I'm not naming products here, but contact me if you want some recommendations for green superfood products.)

I highly recommend fasting. If going right into a water fast for several days feels like too much for you, feel free to start with one of the alternative fasts. You can always add a day or more of pure water fasting in the middle of a modified fast.

Look at your fast as a new beginning; of launching yourself into a higher level of good health and better eating choices. Fasting may not be for everyone, but for me it was a huge reset in all the four pillars of my health. ☑

When you fast, do not look somber
as the hypocrites do, for they disfigure their faces
to show others they are fasting... But when you fast,
put oil on your head and wash your face,
so that it will not be obvious to others
that you are fasting, but only to your Father,
who sees what is done in secret
and will reward you.

—Matthew 16:18

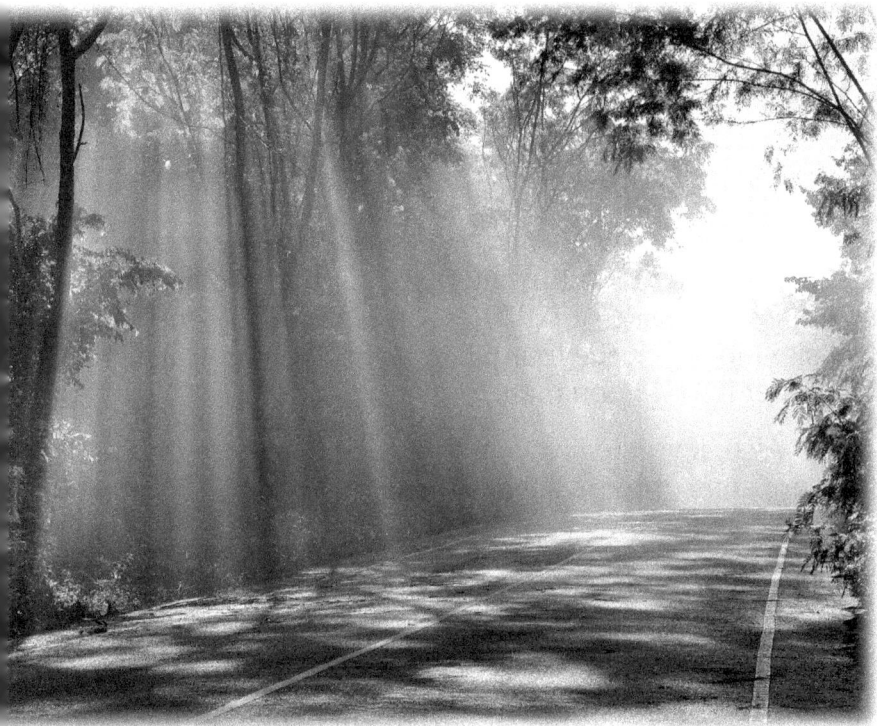

The End of
the Beginning

THE END OF THE BEGINNING—
Just Getting Started

WOW, you stuck with me to the end! Don't stop here, my friend! I want to help you on your personal journey to great health—discovering that life mission of yours and living your life in a way that is healthy, full of passion and purpose.

Next steps would be to begin to get my newsletter, where you will be on the cutting edge of men's health. Sign up on my website: The4PillarsOfMensHealth.com. On my website I focus on the four pillars—check out my latest blogs and other information there.

Also, if you really want to go deep on these four pillars here are some intense suggestions:

PILLAR #1—Accurate Thinking

Napoleon Hill is one of the founding fathers of positive, healthy, and therefore, more accurate thinking. He spent 20 years interviewing the most successful people in the United States at the beginning of the 20th century. People like Thomas Edison, Henry Ford and Dale Carnegie. He was able to synthesis a system of thinking that has produced incredible results in me and many others. All his books are great reads, but the Napoleon Hill Foundation has an intense course you should check out if you're interested in major growth. [Find it at: Naphill.org/get-involved/why-get-certified/.]

PILLAR #2—Nutrition

If you want more information on nutrition and how it affects your body and life, I recommend Dr. Fuhrman's Nutritarian Education Institute. It is one of the best investments

I made in myself. Not only did I learn about how nutrition effects my life, but it also cemented in my soul the importance of eating well. You can find it at DrFuhrman.com/learn/nutritarian-education-institute.

PILLAR #3—Exercise

It's important to find a type of exercise that you love and that you will stick with. If you're interested in what makes my heart sing in this area, check out my self-challenge to run all 723 miles of the magnificent trails along the Absaroka-Beartooth Wilderness at Run723.com.

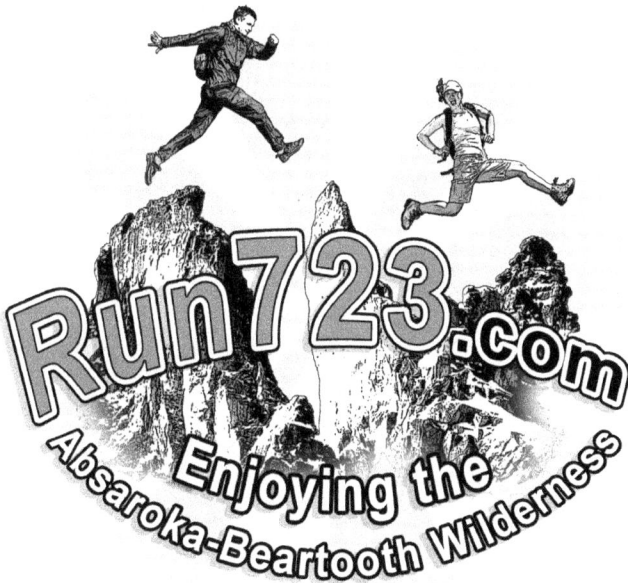

PILLAR #4—Spirituality

Digging deep into your spiritual being is amazing!! Get involved with some like-minded people who are committed to growing in this area of life. The camaraderie will help you grow spiritually and socially.

I am all about growing. If you have any comments, questions or suggestions, I would love to hear from you. I hope to meet you some day and swap stories of GREAT HEALTH! ☑

Lets stay in touch!

Send correspondence by email to

the4pillarsofmenshealth@gmail.com

or by snail mail via

PINE CREEK PUBLISHING HOUSE
P.O. Box 833
Livingston, Montana 59047

Copies of this book can be ordered at

Amazon.com

or from my website:

The4PillarsOfMensHealth.com

where you can also get my latest
updates on health and well-being.

Follow our treks through the
Absaroka-Beartooth Wilderness at

Run723.com

ABOUT THE AUTHOR

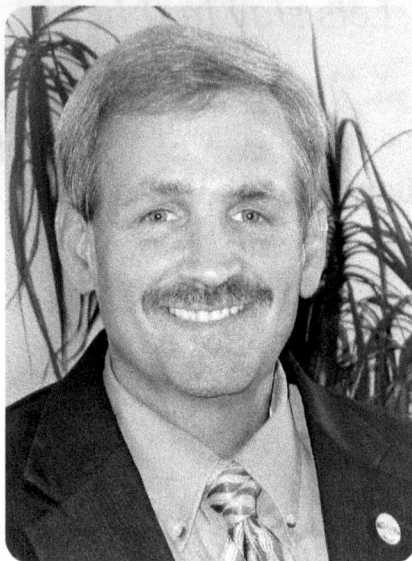

Dave Skattum is a family man, a health guru and an inspirational speaker. He is also a business entrepreneur, a youth pastor, a Distinguished Toastmaster, a Certified Nutritarian, and a Certified Napoleon Hill Foundation Instructor.

In his late forties, some life-changing experiences created a starting gate for Dave to make drastic changes in his life, and started him on his quest to improve his overall health and well-being. Since then, he has taken off 70 pounds, participates in Triathlons and Ultra Trail Running, has weaned himself off junk food, and enjoys nutritious foods and periodic fasting. In addition, he has become accurate and more positive in his thinking, and has taken his spiritual life to a new level.

These four lifestyle upgrades he calls *The 4 Pillars of Men's Health*. He now brings excitement and hope to audiences when speaking or blogging about his journey to achieving and maintaining great health and wellness.

www.ingramcontent.com/pod-product-compliance
Lightning Source LLC
Chambersburg PA
CBHW062055270326
41931CB00013B/3086